The Agony of Obesity

Dr. Judith Giustini

Contents

1. Introduction

By: Dr. Judith Giustini

This book started out to be a few encouraging hand-outs to provide my pudgy patients with some useful information from one who has been in "The Battle of the Bulges" since age 12. Obesity is such a complicated topic because there are so many ways to get there, considering our complicated lifestyles, our unresolved subconscious negative feelings, our habits, and our lack of knowledge about diet and nutrition.

If you have been dealing with the mean and evil Obesity Monster for "a while", you know that you need all the help you can get, but sometimes, you are so discouraged that you don't want to even try (again!) to be a normal-weight person. You need scientific knowledge – how many calories you need to consume each day, what happens if you consume too many calories (you gain 1 lb. if you consume 3,500 calories more than you burn, no matter how long it takes) and how many calories you can consume per day if you choose to lose 2 lbs. per week (1,200 for a woman and 1,500 for a man). You also need compassion, understanding, and encouragement.

If you are in a state of exasperation and some negative feelings about yourself, you do not need a book that is all complicated and contains a bunch of terminology you don't understand. That is why the chapters in this book are about 250-350 words each, and intended to be easy to understand.

2. Preface

By: Dr. Judith Giustini

<u>How did you get fat?</u>
Were you an obese child?
What kinds of food did you eat when you were young?
Did you gain the "Freshman 20" at college?
Did you gain the "COVID 19" during the Pandemic?
What kinds of food do you eat now?
Do you eat at home, at work? In restaurants?
How much weight are you looking to lose?
What weight loss methods have you tried before?
How did that work out for you?
Fat is fat, but everybody's story is different.

In this book you will find information about your internal organs, scientific tests of the pH of your saliva and urine, and the 5-Hour Glucose Tolerance Test, 26 stresses that interfere with dieting success, recipes for Super Soup and Super Shakes, and some calories in foods.

If you have a lot of weight to lose, it is going to take you a long time to recuperate from this sickness of obesity that you have brought upon yourself. It would be so easy to just give up right in the middle of things (again?). But NOW you have this book. Every page is a chapter – not too much to read, but something to think about, on your favorite subject: your health, happiness, and success. Maybe you can read one or two chapters each day, and keep your mind on your goal of living in a normal-weight body. Think what a good example you will become to your friends and relations who may be struggling with the same dilemma. Can you request Divine assistance?

3. A Diet That Works

By: Dr. Judith Giustini

You have some weight to lose. Too bad about those food and drink choices that landed you in this situation. They are *not* your friends, but it's still going to be difficult to say bye to them. Maybe you have tried many different methods to get your weight under control – high protein diets, diet pills, stomach stapling, and you are still in the struggle with the Evil Obesity Monster. NEWS FLASH: You can't keep doing what you were doing to cause the problem and expect a different result. Why did you eat and drink those things? Maybe you ate what you ate because you liked what you liked. You can do better.

Maybe nobody told you that you would gain weight if you ate more than 2,500 calories per day (man) or 2,000 (woman). A drive thru burger could be 550 calories, a medium shake 500 calories and a medium order of fries 350 calories. That's 1,400 calories for lunch. What are you going to eat the rest of the day? Worse: these foods are not very nutritious, and that feeling of fullness may be gone in 2 hr. Even worse: You ae not providing the trillions of cells in your body that are working to keep you alive with the nutrients they need to do a good job.

You are not fat because you don't like to eat. Many weight loss diets feature a plan where you still eat the foods that made you fat, only in smaller portions, so you are going to go around hungry. There is a whole world of fruits and vegetables who can become your new friends. They will help you lose weight, and they will help your cells to keep you alive. See: Ch. 8., Ch. 41. Ch. 162. and Ch. 163.)

4. A "Normal" Day of What You Eat

By: Dr. Judith Giustini

Skipping breakfast may seem like a good idea at the time, because you had a big dinner the night before, and you are not very hungry in the morning. There will be no dishes to wash before work, and just think of all those breakfast calories you won't be eating. Hey, maybe you will lose some weight. But by skipping breakfast, you are setting yourself up for a yo-yo blood sugar situation, where what you eat will be a dominant feature of your day and evening.

By mid-morning, your blood sugar is low, and you are cranky and irritable. After a donut (250 cal.) and some coffee with cream and sugar (150 cal.), you are in a better mood, and you go back to work.

By lunchtime, you are hungry again, and you gobble down a big burger (550 cal.), a vanilla shake (500 cal.) and some fries (350 cal.). By mid-afternoon, your energy is getting low, so you have a soda (12 oz. 150 cal.) and chips (300 cal.).

At dinner, you have 2 glasses of wine (5 fl. ounces 123 cal. x 2 =246 cal. a roll with butter (200 cal.), a salad with creamy dressing (200 cal.), a baked potato (110 cal), 2 Tbs. sour cream (46 cal.) 6-oz. steak (400 cal.) and some broccoli (60 cal.). At bedtime, you have a little dish of chocolate ice cream (200 cal.), and your grand total of calories for the day is 3,749, *and* you may not be hungry for breakfast, so you will start the same scenario over again.

5. You Can Choose a Different Diet

By: Dr. Judith Giustini

A normal-weight woman burns about 2,000 calories per day. That's 2,500 calories per day for a man. To the person in Ch. 4. A "Normal" Day of What You Eat, it probably didn't *seem* as if they were overeating – certainly not pigging out. If you overeat by 100 calories per day (3,500 calories), you will gain about 1 lb. per month. To lose that 1 lb., you will need to "un-eat 3,500 calories).

If you choose to lose about 2 lb. per month, you will need to limit your daily calorie intake to 2,000 for a woman and 2,500 for a man. You will have to say good-bye to junk foods donuts, chips, French fries, sodas with sugar, shakes, if you choose to drink alcohol, you need to count the calories.

In the example in Ch. 4., the person consumed 3,749 calories, and about 1,900 of them were junk foods. Delete the junk foods, and that leaves about 1,849 "good" calories – not "Nutritionally Aware" (Ch. 161.) calories, and maybe the person would have felt "deprived" or still hungry without them. Junk foods are a money-making scheme. What's in them? What are those words on the label?

You have to live in this body for the rest of your life. It is so easy to gain weight, and Obesity is no darn fun. If you choose to live in a normal-weight body for the rest of your life, you are going to have to choose a different diet.

6. Alkaline Diet for Health

By: Dr. Judith Giustini

Authorities on nutrition and health have said that that every disease flourishes in an acid body. Foods that leave an acid ash after they are burned in the body are grains and high protein foods such as animal flesh, fish and dairy products.

Most fruits and vegetables are alkaline-ash foods. Raw fruits and vegetables contain enzymes that help digest them. They also contain vital nutrients in a form that is naturally usable by your cells. You can use it to balance your blood sugar and lose weight. Ideally, it should be 80% fruits and vegetables and 20% other nutrients. It is important to drink enough water for yourself – at least 64 oz. per day. You can learn to test and understand the meaning of your urine pH.

A simple way to work fruits and vegetables into your diet is "The Super Shakes Plan", which contains eggs, milk, fruits and vegetables plus Stevia. You need a blender. You don't have to peel most of the fruits. Try some vegetables, such as raw squash and cauliflower and cooked beans and sweet potatoes.

If you have been living on "Typical American Diet", you may have been doing "Starvation in the Midst of Plenty". The Super Shakes Plan provides Nutrient-Dense Nutrition. For weight loss: 1,200 calories/day for a woman, 1,500 for a man.

7. The Alkaline Weight Loss Diet

By: Dr. Judith Giustini

How did you get fat? You got fat by consuming more calories than you burned. What have you been eating? Fruits and vegetables leave an "alkaline ash" after they are burned in your body, and it is easy for your body to get rid of. Proteins leave an "acid ash", and it is more difficult for your body to get rid of.

An alkaline diet is a plant-based diet that will allow you to eat plenty of food, so you never feel hungry or deprived. Fruits and vegetables provide vital nutrients that are not available in the fast food you get at the drive-up window. A plant-based diet contributes to your long-term wellness. Brown rice and beans are somewhat acid, but they supply many nutrients and add to satiety.

Changing to a plant-based diet can seem like a big job or a fun adventure. Since you are going to need to be on it for the rest of your life, it would be in your best interest to take on a good attitude. You don't have to do this alone. The books of Dr. Joel Fuhrman will help you. Some weight loss groups are into diet pills these days. Is this what you want for your long-term health?

According to Dr. F. Batmanghelidj, in *Your Body's Many Cries for Water,* chronic dehydration is a major cause of obesity. Many doctors and weight-loss groups recommend 64 ounces of water per day.

8. About Your New Lifestyle

By: Dr. Judith Giustini

Your lifestyle involves the Six Essentials": what you eat, drink, and breathe, and how you exercise, rest, and think. You might presume that these are choices you make with your conscious mind on an "as-needs" basis, but really, they are running on programming that was established in your subconscious mind way back when. They are now part of your belief system, and you are kind of on "autopilot".

If you choose to make a change in what you eat or drink, you are going to have to deal with your belief system, and it is like a stern parent who is in charge of how things should be and ought to be. Your conscious mind is 10% of your thinking, and your subconscious mind is 90% of your thinking. Your puny little conscious mind will have to do battle with your gigantic subconscious mind.

Chapter 117. is "Why is it So Difficult to Change Your Habits?" You might have to contend with your habits on a millisecond-to-millisecond basis, day in and day out for "a while" before you can give your new lifestyle choice a new home in your belief system. Even so, there is a tendency for "backsliding". You might have to keep talking to yourself and disciplining yourself day in and day out.

Whenever you make a change in one of The Six Essentials, it affects many other things in your life. If you change what you eat, it can require you to change where you have lunch and with whom. If you change what you drink, it might affect how you spend your time in the evenings or on weekends. You can take charge of things in your life.

9. Type 2 diabetes

By: Dr. Judith Giustini

webmd.com says that type 2 diabetes is "a lifelong disease that keeps your body from using insulin the way it should". After you eat, your body converts your food to glucose which is meant to be used in your cells for energy. Insulin is a hormone made by your pancreas When you have type 2 diabetes, your cells do not open up to receive the glucose, so it builds up in your blood.

Some symptoms of type 2 diabetes are: hunger even after you have eaten, dry mouth due to dehydration caused by frequent urination, because your kidneys need water to get rid of your excess blood sugar, numbness in your hands or feet, fatigue and slow wound healing.

In his book *You're Not Sick, You're Thirsty,* Dr. F. Batmanghelidjsays that type 2 diabetes is related to chronic cellular dehydration. He recommends drinking no less than two quarts of water daily plus some increased salt intake. He says that this type of diabetes is often reversible. In his book *An Apple a Day – is it Enough Today?* Dr. M. T. Morter, Jr., M.A., D.C. says that one cause of type 2 diabetes is a high protein diet. He says the cells do not want to open up to receive nutrients from the blood, because they are toxic (sick) due to the acid diet. In her book *Feelings Buried Alive Never Die,* Karol K. Truman says that some *"Probable feelings causing illness"* of diabetes are: judging self and others harshly, disappointment in life, and feelings of sorrow.

10. Antioxidants

By: Dr. Judith Giustini

Oxidation is a chemical reaction in the cells of your body that can produce free radicals, which are compounds that can damage your cells and are thought to be involved with premature aging, cancers, and strokes. Back in the 1980's, people were trying to sell pills of "antioxidants" to their friends and relations in multi-level marketing schemes, but very few people knew the meaning of the word *antioxidants*, so this product was not a big seller.

Antioxidants are found in fresh, raw fruits and vegetables. In large clinical trials, antioxidants separated from natural sources did not show any benefits. They need natural co-factors to be used in the body.

Nutritional deficiencies are not the only cause of aging or nervous system breakdown. In her book *Feelings Buried Alive Never Die,* Karol K. Truman says that certain illnesses are linked to certain subconscious negative thinking patterns. For example, Alzheimer's disease patients often have Suppressed anger and Feelings of helplessness and hopelessness. Parkinson's disease patients often have many Fears. The chronic stress of subconscious unresolved negative feelings can overwhelm your organ systems. When things in your body start to break down, you worry about yourself, and this can cause you to break down faster or develop other symptoms. Stress causes illness.

In his book *You're Not Sick, You're Thirsty,* Dr. F. Batmanghelidj explains the relationship between chronic dehydration and the various systems of the body, causing symptoms that are labeled as "Diseases".

11. Are You Addicted to Empty Calories?

By: Dr. Judith Giustini

Fruits, vegetables, beans, brown rice and nuts contain complex molecules that supply valuable nutrients. Your digestive acids and enzymes are made from nutrients in your diet. If your diet is deficient, it won't be able to make them.

Empty calories are made of small molecules that digest rapidly. If you have been living on a diet of white bread, pasta, sugar and alcohol, your body may not have the ability to digest larger molecules. You may seem to be addicted to empty calorie foods, because they may be all you are able to digest.

Small molecules from grains, sugar, and alcohol elevate your blood sugar Your pancreas secretes insulin to bring it down, but when your pancreas becomes stressed from overuse, it does not respond as quickly to elevated blood sugar and it may delay in secreting insulin, then secrete too much at one time. This can result in your blood sugar going too low, which will mean your brain is starving for sugar, causing you to grab anything sweet to eat.

When you live on empty calories, your general state of health is going to decline, because you are treating your blood sugar emergency and missing out on vital nutrients. Your energy level is going to be low. You may resort to stimulants such as caffeine, tobacco, alcohol, prescription medications or street drugs to keep your energy up. This is a good way to make an old person out of a young person.

12. Are You an Apple or a Pear?

By: Dr. Judith Giustini

From Internet sources:

You have an apple-shaped body if you have abdominal obesity. People who have this body type tend to have more heart disease, diabetes, and strokes. Apple-shaped people have higher levels of insulin, fatty acids, cholesterol, and blood pressure.

If you have a pear-shaped body, your extra weight is in your buttocks and thighs. Pear-shaped people are seen to have more varicose veins, which is thought to be due to fat compressing the veins of the lower body, and blocking it from returning to the heart.

In his book *Body Shape Diets,* Dr. Eric Berg shows sketches of and discusses 4 main body types:

THE THYROID BODY TYPE has excess fat more evenly distributed. Dr. Berg says this patient's body does not produce enough thyroid hormone.

THE ADRENAL BODY TYPE has a "barrel" midsection (fat is a big bulge under the belly button and arms and legs are thin. Dr. Berg says this person's adrenal glands do not work properly.

THE OVARY BODY TYPE has lower body fat- "saddle bags" on the upper thighs, lower stomach, and buttocks. Dr. Berg says this is due to malfunction of the ovaries, and they are producing excess estrogen.

THE LIVER BODY TYPE has a "pot belly". Dr. Berg says this is not fat. It is water. He says that when the liver is not doing well, it leaks water into the stomach area. This swelling feels like a water balloon when you push it.

13. Are You a Nighttime Nibbler?

By: Dr. Judith Giustini

It can be a long time between dinner time and breakfast time. Maybe you have just spent the whole day "being good" on your diet. You surely do not want to undo all your good work by heavy-duty nibbling in the evening. Maybe you are actually hungry, or maybe you are just bored. What can you eat and still stay on your diet?

If you are on The Super Shakes Plan, maybe you have a nice glass of your delicious shake. If your blender jar running a little low in the afternoon, maybe you can add some fruits, milk and Stevia. If you haven't had the rest of your eggs yet, you could put them in your shake, or maybe make a little meal of them. Eggs give you a feeling of satiety.

If you are not on the Super Shakes Plan, but you want to stay on your Calorie Consciousness Program, it's good if you prepare ahead of time. Shop for the kinds of fruits you like. When you get hungry at night, you can have a bowl of your favorite fruits – maybe sprinkle with some Stevia. How about some leftover stir-fry?

Everybody's situation, likes and dislikes are different, but a calorie is still a calorie. If you have gained weight due to consuming excess calories, you are going to have to "un-consume" those calories – better to do it in the most painless way possible. If you have a lot of weight to lose, and you are sticking to the 1,200 – 1,500, you have to count ALL the calories –daytime and nighttime.

14. Are You Obese?

By: Dr. Judith Giustini

If you are obese, you are not alone. The scourge of obesity is spreading around the world.

How did you get fat? That's what the speaker at the weight loss group screamed out at the class members. And then she told us about all the excesses with food that had caused her to be 200 lbs. overweight. She said that she had declared Friday as "Pizza Night", and then she would get on the phone and order 2 large pizzas and drive to the pizza place to pick up the food, even though the pizza place offered free delivery. This was so she could eat one of the pizzas on the way home. She said she also would buy a bag of candy bars and drive around and eat them, throwing the wrappers (evidence) out the window.

Maybe you do not pig-out, but you put extra butter (100 calories per Tbs.) on your potatoes, or you indulge in chocolate candies (read the labels). If you consume 100 calories per day more than you burn for 35 days, you will gain 1 lb.

If losing weight were a simple process, where you merely eat less and exercise more, it would be easier to lose weight. What you eat and drink is influenced by your culture, what's available, addictions, your subconscious belief system, your habits, your feelings, your associations and many other factors. How much you weigh is not a simple number on a scale.

Ch. 168. Feelings Associated with "obesity words.

15. Are You Toxic?

By: Dr. Judith Giustini

Air pollution, coal-burning electrical plants, pharmaceutical drugs in water, oil spills, leaking nuclear waste . . . environmental toxins can make you sick.

Your body is exposed to toxins through what you eat, Chronic dehydration can be a cause of toxicity, because you need water to wash the toxins out of your body.

When you use your mind to criticize, condemn and complain, your body creates toxic chemicals that have great power over your health, happiness, and success and over the type of experiences and relationships you attract into your life.

In her book *Feelings Buried Alive Never Die,* Karol K. Truman lists under *"Probable Feelings Causing Ill-Ness", under "Toxins:* Negative feelings and thoughts against yourself and Giving away your power". In her book, she provides an extensive list of "Ill-nesses" and the negative feelings that may be causing them.

In Mind-Body Therapy, you can find out what those feelings are, and you can stop their power over you through forgiving them and replacing them with the specific positive feeling for each one that energetically negate the power of the negative feeling.

This is the step away from Confusion to Clarity (Self-Awareness). The next step is Focus (Self-Knowledge) and after that comes Peace. It can be quite a journey.

16. "There's Nothing So Powerful as an Idea Whose Time Has Come" (a quotation attributed to Albert Einstein)

By: Dr. Judith Giustini

There is a Pandemic of Obesity. Just look around you, or maybe in the mirror?

The ostensible cause of obesity is too many calories. If you consume 3,500 calories more than you burn, nonmatter how long it takes, you will gain 1 lb. To lose that 1 lb., you need to "un-eat" or exercise off those 3,500 calories. The math is simple, but people are complicated.

What if Calorie Consciousness (Ch. 160.) were to become the new Big Idea? The original Weight Watchers diet, from 50 years ago, was 1,200 calories per day for women and 1,500 calories per day for men. This is also the calorie recommendation of a local M.D. who treats obesity patients, and they are required to write down everything they eat and drink.

Calorie Consciousness can be the place where you begin in dealing with this very important influence on your health, happiness, and success. This can lead to Nutritional Awareness (Ch. 161.). Considering the vital importance of this information, it would be nice if we had learned it in grade school.

You can get a lot of information online about the calorie and nutritional content of the foods you buy at the store and the foods on restaurant menus.

17. Beware Fragmented Foods

By: Dr. Judith Giustini

Refined foods are devoid of enzymes, so your body must create the enzymes that are needed to digest them from previously stored material from your diet. White bread, donuts, pizza dough, pasta, many breakfast cereals, candies, corn chips, potato chips, French fries, soda, etc. all contain empty calories. If you think you are eating something nutritious, you are fooling yourself.

Everything you eat or drink needs to be digested. Enzymes and digestive juices are made from the nutrients in your diet. If your diet lacks nutrients, you will eventually have trouble digesting foods. Some foods are more complicated to digest than other foods are. If you lack the ability to digest complicated foods, you are going to be stuck eating fragmented foods because that's all you can digest.

Some people think they can make up for eating empty calories by taking vitamin pills, but this is not true, according to Dr. M. T. Morter, Jr. M.A., D.C., who taught that f you take a high-dosage calcium supplement, for example, the excess calcium depletes the enzymes and cofactors needed to utilize the calcium and your body responds as if there is a deficiency of calcium.

Your body is made up of cells. Each cell is like a little person. It takes in nutrients and excretes wastes. Your cells function best on a plant-based diet of raw foods that supply the enzymes, vitamins and minerals that are needed to digest them. After fruits and vegetables are digested, they leave an alkaline ash, which helps neutralize the acids in your diet that make you toxic.

18. Calories DO Count

By: Dr. Judith Giustini

- Overeat by 100 calories per day, gain 1 lb. in 35 days.

- Males 1,500 Calories, Females 1,200 Calories: lose 2 lbs. in 7 days.

- Assess your present calorie intake. How many/day now?

- Males maintain weight at about 2,500 calories, Females: 2,000.

- Many obese people are hypoglycemic or diabetic. You may need to consume small veggie meals every two hours until your blood sugar becomes stable.

- If you choose a plant-based diet, you can be on a weight loss diet without being hungry. This is important if you have a lot of weight to lose.

- Your diet should be 80% fruits and vegetables and 20% other choices.

- WATER: In his book *Your Body's Many Cries for Water,* Dr. F. Batmanghelidj recommends ½ ounce per day per pound you weigh. A weight loss group says at least 64 oz. per day

- EXERCISE: if you are able, not embarrassed to be seen. Start out with walking if you are able to walk. You are the person who eats your food and drinks your beverages, so you are the person who can stop eating and drinking the things that made you fat.

19. Carbohydrates

By: Dr. Judith Giustini

The term *carbohydrate* refers to organic compounds that consist of carbon, hydrogen and oxygen. In biochemistry, *carbohydrate* is another term for saccharide, which is comes from a Greek word. Cellulose from the cell wall of plants is said to be the most abundant organic molecule on earth.

Carbohydrates have been classified as simple carbohydrates or complex carbohydrates. Complex carbohydrates are those found in whole foods such as fruits, vegetables, beans, brown rice, and whole grains, which are foods where fiber, vitamins and minerals are also found. Processed carbohydrates such as pasta, white bread, children's breakfast cereals, corn chips, potato chips, candy, sugary drinks, jams, jellies, alcoholic beverages, pastry, and white rice provide calories, but few other nutrients.

The Food and Agriculture Organization and World Health Organization have recommended that people should get about 55 to 75% of food energy from complex carbohydrates and only 10% from sugars.

If you ae on a weight loss diet, or even if you just want to "eat healthy", you are going to be looking for foods that supply good quality nutrients, contribute to a feeling of fullness and satiety and contribute to alkalinity in your pH. You will find that your best choices are amongst the complex carbohydrate foods such as fruits, vegetables brown rice and beans.

20. Carbohydrates Are Not Evil

By: Dr. Judith Giustini

If you are on a plant-based diet, you will be using lots of carbohydrates. Fruits, vegetables brown rice, beans and whole grains are complete foods. White rice, sugar and white flour are fragmented foods. They require co-factors from the whole foods you eat to process them. Excess use of sugar can lead to hypoglycemia, which is very unpleasant and can lead to type 2 diabetes, which is terrible.

Persons who have diabetes often have high blood cholesterol, high blood pressure, heart disease, kidney disease and arthritis. They are more susceptible to viruses.

Six out of ten of the major causes of death in the U.S. are connected with nutrition. It is in your best interest to learn about the nutritional content of foods and to choose the ones that are good for your health, even though some empty calorie foods are more fun.

Dehydration is a major cause of many chronic degenerative diseases. In his book *Your Body's Many Cries for Water*, Dr. F. Batmanghelidj says we need to drink ½ ounce of water per day for every pound we weigh, plus 1 tsp. of sea salt per gallon of water.

If what you eat and drink are causing your body to try to function without the vital nutrients it needs to thrive, it will do the best it can to keep you alive, but eventually this system and that system will become compromised and you will be in a general run-down condition called exhaustion, which is a stepping-stone on the path to the nursing home.

21. Some Cases of Obesity (1)

By: Dr. Judith Giustini

When a Rhode Island woman was 30 years old, she became the mother of twins. Before she became a mom, she used to run marathons. Between races, she would run many miles per week to train for marathons and she was able to consume many calories per day without gaining weight.

After the twins were born and she was a stay-at-home mom, she kept eating according to her old diet and gained 100 lbs. All the homemaker chores, plus the childcare duties, were over whelming, and she became cranky and argumentative with her husband. She was no longer interested in sex. She felt overburdened and sought refuge in chardonnay. By the time the twins were in kindergarten, she was obese, alcoholic, divorced and distraught.

She became a Mind-Body Therapy patient and started taking charge of things in her life as she moved from Confusion (Yankin' & Crankin') to Clarity (Self-Awareness). she began to take charge of things in her life. She joined a weight loss group and joined a gym. She was able to discontinue using alcohol, which was a major component of her calorie intake each day.

Eventually, she got her weight down to where it was before her pregnancy. The twins are in college now, and she has met the new love of her life.

22. Some Cases of Obesity (2)

By: Dr. Judith Giustini

A man from a small town in Massachusetts was 55 years old, and he weighed 350 lbs. He was 5'5" tall. His seven younger brothers and sisters had all married and left home, but this man, who was considered to be mildly retarded, was still living with mom and dad.

He was very attached to his mother, who was the person who prepared the meals he enjoyed so much. From the way his father treated him, it seemed that his father was not too pleased that this man was still living at home. Despite the summer heat, he assigned his morbidly obese son to mow a large yard and clean up debris at midday. This work would have been strenuous for normal weight person, but for a 350 lb. man with heart trouble, kidney trouble, high blood pressure and diabetes, it was life-threatening. But this obese man did not object, one wonders if he chose to keep the peace with his dad, so as not to cause interference in his connection with his dear mother and her wonderful kitchen.

This man said he regularly snacked on potato chips, soda and candy bars. He said he had been chubby all his life. He seemed to accept himself the way he was, and not be motivated to change. This, combined with his mental retardation, meant that he was not going to be a good candidate for weight loss counseling or Mind-Body Therapy.

23. Some Cases of Obesity (3)

By: Dr. Judith Giustini

A 52-year-old woman in a suburb of Boston had been living-in with her parents for about 16 years. Her parents were both schoolteachers, and they owned a large home on a big piece of property. She did all the cooking, cleaning, shopping, landscaping, housekeeping, and bookkeeping.

She had a boyfriend for a number of years. A few evenings per week, she would make dinner with him and stay overnight. Her portrait was hanging in his parlor. It was a shock to her when she learned that he had the same arrangement with another girlfriend. He would call home during the day and his daughter would switch the portraits.

This woman was 5'2" tall and she weighed 250 lbs. She loved baking cookies and eating them. She ate all the leftover Halloween candy and the goodies left over from the makeup demonstration party at her house when nobody showed up. When she tried to lose weight, she gained weight. Her glaucoma was getting worse. Was it due to the pressure of the fat around her eyeballs?

After her parents retired and her father died, it was just her and her mother. She had a contentious relationship with her mother all her life and she held a lot of negative feelings towards her. There was a lot of bickering and nibbling food. Her condition of "Fat" was linked to hidden anger towards her brothers, who were favored by her mom.

24. Some Cases of Obesity (4)

By: Dr. Judith Giustini

A 60-Year-Old woman injured her neck and low back in an accident at work, when she fell onto a wheelie desk chair, and it went flying and crashed into some boxes of files and she fell off.

During the course of her care, she kept gaining weight. Both of her knees were bone-on bone, in need of replacements, and the extra lbs. we're causing even more pain.

This woman always seemed to be cranky about something. She was presently living with a man she considered not to be up to the speed of her2nd husband, the undercover agent. She and her boyfriend had purchased a house together, and he was all "honey and sweetheart", and she was all, "Get outta here".

In her book *Feelings Buried Alive Never Die*, Karol K. Truman gives a list of *"Probable Feelings Causing Ill-ness"*. These seem to fit this patient. For *"**Back – Lower**"* it is: "In a relationship that hurts" and for *"**Neck Problems**"* she lists: "non-acceptance & rejection of others". These feelings were related to her father, her uncle, her 2 former husbands, her current boyfriend,

Staying home for a year, she slipped into nibbling. If her boyfriend saw her eating a cookie and said something about it, she would eat 2 more, just for spite. She gained 100 lbs., but she was too distraught to think about doing anything about it.

25. Some Cases of Obesity (5)

By: Dr. Judith Giustini

A 40-year-old woman was homeless in Laguna Beach, California. She and her boyfriend had a storage unit where they kept their stuff. In this area, some people had built $10,000,000homes on a precipice above the ocean. The beach was about 50' below the edge of the cliff. After dark, this homeless couple would get their bedding out of hiding and sleep at the base of the cliff.

This woman kept herself up rather well, considering the circumstances. She had beautiful long blonde hair, and she wore nice long dresses. Pretty spiffy for a 307 lb. lady walking around with a roll of toilet paper in her bag.

Her boyfriend would go to the children's beach each day play "Puff the Magic Dragon" on his guitar and mothers would give their little kids money to toddle up and drop into his open guitar case.

These were complicated people. Lots of negative feelings towards their families. The woman had left home when she was 14. At one point she was living in a Volkswagen bus with her infant. When the bus broke down and the police had it towed, she was out on the street, and the Social Services department had her baby placed in foster care. She suppressed her negative feelings behind chocolate candy.

Her condition of "Overweight" was linked to negative feelings towards the police. Her boyfriend's frequent low back pain was linked to feelings of sadness towards his father, but we didn't get into any serious MBT work.

26. Some Cases of Obesity (6)

By: Dr. Judith Giustini

I was at the YMCA in an exercise class that was being held in the basketball court in the interest of "social distancing" due to the COVID-19Pandemic. Looking up, I saw an enormous man on the walking track above the basketball court. I left the class and went up to find him. His name was Earl, and he weighed 407 lbs.

I invited him to a free weight-loss consultation at my office, where I discussed his health situation and gave him some pages from my book to read. I thought he would be a great case to study, and report on his success with the AOO program.

He was unable to keep working at the tire factory because of his obesity, so he was on some kind of aid program, and his insurance paid for his visits to Duke hospital. He had a heart deliberator and a pacemaker. He had a cyst of water on his abdomen that needed surgery, but not at his current weight.

It was a little bit difficult to get him to focus on what I was trying to tell him, so I just asked him to send me emails of whatever he ate and drank throughout the day. One day, he said he had 2 breakfast sandwiches (450 calories each) and a 40-oz soda (425 calories), for a total of 1,325 calories for breakfast alone.

I wanted him to come to my office once a week, so I could do some educational work with him, but he kept having to be someplace else – in the hospital about his defibrillator or on a trip with his friends. Conclusion: He was no tready to deal with this problem, so I said bye bye.

27. Some Cases of Obesity (7)

By: Dr. Judith Giustini

A 310 lb. woman from Rhode Island was losing sensation in and control of her feet. The condition was beginning to affect her knees as well. She had been to medical doctors and chiropractors about this, with no change in symptoms.

At 45 years of age, she had been the office manager of a large law firm in Providence for ten years. She took her job seriously and often worked overtime. To save time shopping and cooking, she would often eat at fast food places three meals per day.

She was the second oldest of 8 children. Her father had managed to sexually abuse all of them. After she left home, he would visit her at her apartment, demanding sex, and if she refused, he would threaten to abuse her brother, who was still living at home. A social worker found out about her father, and he escaped to California with his wife and the two younger children and, avoided being arrested.

This woman was distraught about her physical condition. There was a slump in the economy and the law firm was not doing well financially. Despite her devotion to her job, there was a chance that she was going to be laid off from work. At the time, there was not much printed information about Mind-Body Therapy and it was difficult for her to understand that the stress of negative feelings was involved with her physical symptoms.

She went back to her chiropractor and I did not see her anymore.

28. Cases of Obesity (8)

By: Dr. Judith Giustini

At 50, a Massachusetts woman weighed 285 lbs. She was the oldest of quite a few siblings. During her childhood, her family lived in a regular size house trailer. Her mother was a stay-at-home mom, and her father was an alcoholic/gambler who worked in a factory. Sometimes, there was no money for food. When the children got older her mother got a job doing housework, and oldest daughter took over the job of mom. The trailer was crowded, so she stayed at her grandmother's and came to work at her mom's place.

Now in her 50's she was on her second marriage, which was to a man she loved, but could not live with, because of his penchant for rum and cigars. She moved into an apartment building she owned, and embarked on a series of Mind-Body Therapy sessions that brought her from Confusion to Clarity, Focus and Peace. She took charge of things in her life. She was able to get her weight down to 170 lbs., and she opened her home to 3 children from her church, whose mother was a drug addict and could not care for them. Because of her history caring for her siblings, a busy household with 3 teenagers seemed kind of "normal" for her. She was a good mentor for the children because she had already let go of her emotional baggage and she had learned to provide a healthy diet for them.

29. Some Cases of Obesity (9)

By: Dr. Judith Giustini

A woman in a small town in Massachusetts was he fourth of the six children of her parents. Her mother stayed home with the children while her father went to work. Hewes an alcoholic, and he would often come home drunk and in a mean mood. When the children would see the lights of his car in the driveway, they would flee to their bedrooms to avoid being yelled at and beaten.

At 50, this woman was married to a nice man and their two sons were grown, but still living at home. She had been struggling with her bodyweight for many years. She had a lot of subconscious negative feelings related to adverse childhood experiences. Her workday ended at 3 PM, and she would go home and prepare a nice meal, and enjoy eating it with her family. On her way home, she would often stop at the burger and ice cream restaurant, and consume a full meal.

Her husband had expressed interest in her having a slimmer body and she kept saying she was trying. However, subconsciously, the extra bodyweight was a symbol of power and desire to throw her weight around. Unfortunately, this feeling was buried beneath a lifetime of other negative feelings that would need to be dealt with first, and she kind of enjoyed her pudgy body and the presence she felt it provided.

She developed diabetes, hypertension, heart trouble and bad knees, but she still could not lose weight, because she could not let go of feeling good about being fat.

30. Some Cases of Obesity (10)

By: Dr. Judith Giustini

A few years ago, there were several "fat shows" on TV. On one show, a 450 lb. man said that he ate when he was happy and ate when he was sad. His youth had been troubled, and he had a lot of unresolved issues. He had lost the feeling in his feet due to diabetes. His occupation was musician. If he lost feeling in his hands, he would be unable to play his guitar. He was motivated to lose weight, but his obesity was linked to a feeling of needing to protect his body and this had to be resolved before he could take charge of thigs in his life and let go of his cushion of fat.

On another show, there was a 700 lb. teenager who was confined to a facility where his food intake was limited. He needed to lose 300 lbs. before he could be a candidate for bypass surgery. We saw him begging and pleading with his mother to take him home. His mom was pretty chubby herself, and home was not going to be a good place for him to lose weight. His condition of "Fat" was linked to a feeling of hidden anger. We did not get to see how his case turned out because it was not on the TV show.

A male person who weighs 300 lbs. needs to consume about 5,000 calories per day to maintain his weight. According to the math, a 700 lb. guy would need to consume at least10,000 calories per day to keep his weight up. To lose one pound, he would have to consume 3,500 calories fewer than those needed to maintain his weight. If he only cut down to 5,000 calories per day, he would lose weight fairly quickly at first. Future episodes probably kept track of his progress. Hopefully, he learned to live on fewer calories per day.

31. Some Cases of Obesity (11)

By: Dr. Judith Giustini

A 30-year-old man in Boston weighed 400 lbs. Back when he was playing semi-pro football, he used to work out at the gym and go running for exercise, in addition to training with his team members and he weighed 250 lbs. Still kind of heavy, but it served him well on the football field. After he injured his knee in a game, and he needed four operations on it, his exercise was limited to limping from the sofa to the refrigerator.

His extra weight was a strain on his knees, and he wanted to lose weight so he could get some kind of job. He signed up with a weight loss group and he followed the diet and attended the meetings. He began to lose 2 lbs. per week and when he got his weight down to 350 lbs., he was able to get a job at an electronics store, watching the monitors of the surveillance cameras. He was able to sit on a stool part of the time and he continued meeting with his weight loss group. At the end of the first year, he had lost 100 lbs. and he was determined to lose another 100 lbs. the next year.

32. Some Cases of Obesity (12)

By: Dr. Judith Giustini

A 42-year-old man had been driving semi-trucks long distances for 20 years. When he first started driving, he weighed 165 lbs. Now he weighed 365 lbs. His back was aching, his energy was low, and he had high blood pressure and diabetes.

Driving a big -rig limited his choice of restaurants. He fell into the habit of eating at fast food places and truck stops.

If you merely consume 100 calories per day more than you burn, you will gain one pound in 35 days. 100 calories would be about ¼ of a medium order of French fries. He also was not getting much exercise, and walking, even a short distance, was exhausting.

Rather than let his fat defeat him, he decided to take charge of things in his life. He went to an RV store and got a kitchenette setup for the back of his truck, and he rigged up a little gym on the side of his truck. In the morning, he would do his stretching and weight-lifting. In the evening, he would walk around the truck stop. If the weather was bad in the morning, he would move his weights into the trailer and exercise in there. If the weather was bad at night, he would get out his little exercise bicycle and ride it in the back of his truck or under a tarp "porch" he had rigged up with a tarp. He would shop at a grocery store before each trip and prepare healthy meals for himself, keeping track of his calories.

It took two years for him to lose 200 lbs. at 2 lbs. per week. Back at 165 lbs., people who had not seen him for a while barely recognized him, and his wife was no longer embarrassed to be seen with him.

33. Childhood Obesity

By: Dr. Judith Giustini

According to the 2014 American Heart Association post online, about 1/3 of US children are overweight or obese (Google says it's over 60%). This condition is related to unhealthy dietary choices and lack of exercise.

Many obese children have high blood pressure, type 2 diabetes, and high cholesterol. Childhood obesity predisposes one to be an obese adult and a sickly person throughout their life.

Some causes of childhood obesity are two-earner families who are pressed for time, so cooking at home can be inconvenient and fast-foods are readily available (although maybe not so cheap anymore). Convenience stores are located near schools. Some kids consume 2-3 lbs. of sugar per week. Empty calories do not support brain function. Caffeine in soda is addictive and dehydrating. Dehydration is linked to autism, ADHD, obesity, depression, diabetes, heart trouble and high blood pressure, which now occur in children as well as adults.

According to Dr. F. Batmanghelidj (watercure.com and *Obesity, Cancer, Depression* book), each person needs ½ ounce of water per day per pound of bodyweight, (plus 1 tsp. of sea salt per gallon of water), so, fat kids need more water. Some schools lack access to water bubblers, and physical education classes have been eliminated, due to lack of funding.

34. Cholesterol

By: Dr. Judith Giustini

Cholesterol is a fat-like substance found in nearly all living animal cells such as liver, brain and nerve tissues. It is also found in blood, bile and many hormones.

The membrane surrounding each cell is about 13% cholesterol. Cholesterol plays a role in changing food into energy and converting the ultraviolet rays of the sun into Vitamin D. Cholesterol is essential to life.

Elevated blood cholesterol levels have been noted in patients who have coronary heart disease. This could be due to excessive fat intake, improper fat metabolism or dehydration.

Dr. F. Batmanghelidj (*Your Body's Many Cries for Water*) says that the body uses cholesterol as a kind of "clay" to protect the cells against dehydration and drought. He says that elevated blood cholesterol is a sign of dehydration. If you are dehydrated, your blood may become more concentrated, thus causing elevated cholesterol.

Dr. Batmanghelidj says, "Chronic cellular dehydration painfully and prematurely kills. Its initial outward manifestations have been until now labeled as "diseases of unknown origin."

Your body's main job is to keep you alive. It needs water for digestion, blood, etc. If you are dehydrated, it has to rob water from one area to help you survive in another area. Your blood contains water. If your body taps this water to keep you from dying, the amount of cholesterol per ml. is going to rise.

35. Creation Story
From Online, author unknown

By: Dr. Judith Giustini

In the beginning God created the heavens and the earth and populated the earth with broccoli, cauliflower, spinach, green, yellow and red vegetables of all kinds so that man and woman would live long and healthy lives. Then, using God's great gifts, Satan created Ben and Jerry's Ice Cream and Krispy Crème Donuts. And Satan said, "You want chocolate with that?" And the man said, "Yes!" and the woman said, "as long as you're at it, add some sprinkles." And they gained 10 pounds and Satan smiled.

And God created the healthful yogurt that the woman might keep the figure that the man found so fair. And Satan brought forth white flour from the wheat and sugar from the cane and combined them and the woman went from size 6 to size 14. So God said, "Try my fresh green salad." And Satan presented Thousand Island dressing, buttery croutons and garlic toast on the side. And the man and woman unfastened their belts following the repast.

God then said, "I have brought you heart-healthy vegetables and olive oil in which to cook them." And Satan brought forth deep fried fish and chicken-fried steak so big it needed its own platter. And the man gained more weight and his cholesterol went through the roof. God then created a light, fluffy white cake, named it Angel Food Cake, and said, "It is good." Satan then created chocolate cake and named it "Devil's Food."

God then brought forth running shoes so that His children might lose those extra pounds. And Satan gave cable TV with a remote control so Man would not have to toil changing the channels. And Man and Woman laughed and cried before the flickering blue channels and gained pounds.

Then God brought forth the potato, naturally low in fat and brimming with nutrition. And Satan peeled off the healthful skin and sliced the starchy center into chips and deep-fried them. And Man gained pounds. God then gave lean beef so that Man might consume fewer calories and still satisfy his appetite. And Satan created McDonald's and its 99-cent double cheeseburger. Then Satan said, "You want fries with that?" and man replied, "Yes! And supersize them!" And Satan said, "It is good" and Man went into cardiac arrest. God sighed and created quadruple bypass surgery.

36. Creeping Weight Gain

By: Dr. Judith Giustini

37

If you overeat by 3,500 calories, you will gain a pound. To lose that pound, you have under-eat by or exercise off 3.500 calories. The heavier you are, the more calories you have to eat to keep from losing weight.

Maybe you just had an extra soda (160 calories) or an extra order of fries (350 calories, plus the ketchup calories). It is so easy to consume more calories than you burn, and so difficult to consume fewer calories than it takes to maintain your weight. Your weight can gradually creep up and you will be a fattie, even if you are not a glutton.

If you overeat at a holiday meal and give your body more food than it can process at the present time, it tends to store the extra calories as fat.

A man who weighs 360 lbs. said that he has been gaining 10 lbs. per year for the past 10 years. He said he had been working out at a gym (scary). A man his size should be careful to keep his pulse below 120.

A woman in Connecticut had trouble with her weight all her life. Now, at 45 years old, she weighed 280 lbs. After her gastric bypass surgery, she lost weight, but as she started adding candy, soda and alcohol her weight started creeping back up.

37. Defensive Dining

By: Dr. Judith Giustini

If you are obese, eating what you like has placed you at risk for early death. You will definitely lose weight on a diet of 1,200 calories per day (for women) or 1,500 calories per day (for men). If you consume 500 fewer calories than you burn each day for 7 days, you will lose 2 lbs.

Before you start your diet, go through your house, and throw away all the food and beverage items you should not be eating or drinking. Ask your family members can keep their snacks out of your reach. Defensive dining means you plan ahead for circumstances that can take you away from your new lifestyle.

Go shopping for the foods for your diet: fresh or frozen vegetables, fresh fruits, boneless skinless chicken breast, beans, etc. Prepare your stir-fry, soup or salad. Eat some and save some. Boil some white and/or sweet potatoes and keep them on hand for recipes. Potatoes digest slowly and help you feel satisfied. It's the butter that makes them fattening.

Plan your meals ahead of time. This is a war. You need to get your battle gear up and working. If you have hypoglycemia, be prepared to have appropriate snacks and meals every two hours. You might need a thermos and some hot/cold bags.

Stay on your diet when you eat out. Avoid fast food places. Count every calorie. 5 ounces of wine is 123 calories. 1 ounce of vodka is 65. Your body burns the alcohol first, and stores the food as fat. You can get a good veggie meal in a Chinese restaurant. Order steamed vegetables and brown rice. Resist the temptation to nibble from your friends' dishes.

38. Dehydration

By: Dr. Judith Giustini

In his books, *You're Not Sick, You're Thirsty* and *Your Body's Many Cries For Water,* Dr. F. Batmanghelidj lists conditions such as allergies, asthma, attention deficit disorder, high blood pressure, coronary heart disease, obesity, strokes, Type 2 diabetes, impotence, low libido and many other conditions, as being caused by dehydration. He discusses the physiological reasons for this connection in depth.

Dr. Batmanghelidj says we need to drink ½ ounce of water each day for every pound we weigh, and consume 1 tsp. of sea salt per gallon of water. If you have been drinking very little water for a long time, your kidneys may not be working very well. It is important not to get "hydration religion" and overwhelm your kidneys with water. The water you drink before meals goes into your digestive juices. Two glasses of water ½ hour before each meal is a good place to start.

Dehydration causes an "emergency" in your body that causes it to go into the fight-or-flight mode, where healing is not a priority. Dehydration can be a hidden cause of your health going "downward-mobile".

Dehydration is certainly a major physiological stress that you need to eliminate by taking charge of things in your life. Nothing is as simple as it seems, however. You may also have to consider what foods and other beverages you have been consuming and your subconscious negative thoughts, feelings, beliefs, and memories.

39. Dehydration as a Cause of Stress

By: Dr. Judith Giustini

How do you know if you are dehydrated? Look at your symptoms. Are you obese? Are you constipated? Do you have high blood pressure? Do you have diabetes, arthritis, heart trouble, allergies or asthma? Are you depressed? Is your urine a dark color? Is it smelly? If you have these symptoms, your first thought to remedy them might not be that you need to drink more water.

Dehydration causes physical symptoms, but it also causes an emergency in your body, because it is a life and death situation. Your brain and your kidneys are in constant need of water. You need water for your cardiovascular system and your lymph. You need water for digestive juices and joint spaces. Dehydration is an emergency. Emergencies require your physiology to go into a fight-or flight mode, which is not the healing mode.

When you are dehydrated, your body has to figure out where the need for water is the greatest (what is the most life-threatening situation at the moment) and where it can rob water from to remedy this situation but oops, this other place needs it too. What a mad scramble going on inside of you, just because you didn't drink your water. For your body to be in a state of fight-or-flight requires it to produce stress hormones and neurotransmitters. The whole body has to go on alert. Fight-or flight is supposed to be for a temporary situation, not a chronic emergency. The stress of dehydration can certainly interfere with your body's ability to heal itself.

40. A Dieting Method That Did Not Work

By: Dr. Judith Giustini

A woman in Boston went shopping for clothes, thinking her old ones had shrunk in the dryer. She was surprised to see that the XL's no longer fit her, and she needed 1X and 2X. When she got on the scale, she was surprised to see that she now weighed 200 lbs.

She decided to take charge of her bodyweight by going on a fast. She suffered all day with hunger pangs and mood swings. She said some harsh things to her fellow employees that she hoped they could forgive her for. By evening, she could not wait to get to the all-you-can-eat buffet.

Her new plan was to skip one meal per day. Unfortunately, the meal she decided to eliminate was breakfast. By mid-morning, she was ravenous and all she could find to eat was chips, so she got a soda also. (400 cal.)

For lunch she had a burger (500 cal.), fries (350 cal.) and a soda 200 cal.) By mid-afternoon, she was hungry again, and she did not want to sit in the meeting feeling sleepy and irritable, so she bought a candy bar and a soda from the machines (500 cal.).

At dinner with friends, she had wine (200 cal.), rolls (150 cal.) and butter (200 cal.), soup (150 cal.), salad/dressing (200 cal.) steak (400 cal.), baked potato (150 cal.) and butter (200 cal.). Before bed, she had a dish of chocolate ice crem (300 cal.), for a grand total of about 3,700 calories for the day, about 700 calories more than she needs to maintain her weight of 200 lbs.

41. Divorce Your Old Diet!

By: Dr. Judith Giustini

For years, you have been "married" to a diet that has eventually ended you up with bad effects, such as obesity, which is a gateway to many chronic diseases and negative feelings about yourself.

Back in the day, this diet seemed "Okay" to you. You ate what you ate because you liked what you liked. And then there were the holidays . . . as your weight crept up.

If your relationship with food and drink is no longer comfortable for you, it is not going to get better if you simply ignore it. Changing what you eat and drink is a big deal. Everything affects everything else. Divorcing your old diet is going to be a stress for a while, but the benefits are worth it.

Obesity brings its companions: fatigue, self-loathing, pain in your joints, trouble moving around, high blood pressure, stress on your heart, diabetes, worrying about yourself. Your relationship with your old diet has left you obese and deficient in the vital nutrients your body needs to keep you alive. It has not been kind to you.

You may have tried many times to leave your old diet and ended up falling back into your comfort zone with it and then you were right back in bed with the cause of your obesity.

By now, your organ systems may be on life-support. You are probably dehydrated. You are confused and you lack the correct information to take charge of things in your life. A problem once recognized is half-solved. You may need professional help.

42. Do Not Become Hungry, Angry, Lonely or Tired

By: Dr. Judith Giustini

If you are going on a weight loss program that you will need to be on for a long time, you need to take charge of things in your life.

DO NOT BECOME HUNGRY: If you get hungry, you set yourself up for grabbing anything that's available and eating it quickly. If what you ate is a source of empty calories, you are going to be hungry again in a short while and tomorrow you will not be a happy when you step on the scale. See: "Defensive Dining" (Ch. 37.).

DO NOT BECOME ANGRY: For you to lose weight, your digestive and hormonal systems need to be functioning properly. Anger puts your physiology into the fight-or-flight mode, which is the opposite mode from the mode where you lose weight. Anger wears you out, and it does not attract congenial relationships. Go up in your imaginary helicopter and take a look at your life. Can you choose a different feeling – maybe Compassion or Mercy?

DO NOT BECOME LONELY: Loneliness can lead to a "poor me baby" attitude, a feeling of being insecure or disconnected. These feelings can lead to getting together with your old friends Ben & Jerry and Sarah Lee. If you focus on your loneliness, it will grow.

DO NOT BECOME TIRED: If you are tired, you may skip a trip to the store or the farmers market to get the things you need for your diet. Are you sleeping well? Lack of sleep is connected with gaining weight. Insomnia is connected with feelings of: guilt, fear, anxiety, worry and low self-esteem. Dehydration causes fatigue and interferes with your weight loss diet. See book: *Obesity Cancer Depression* by Dr. F. Batmanghelidj

43. What You Drink as a Cause of Stress that Interferes with Healing

By: Dr. Judith Giustini

In his book *Your Body's Many Cries for Water,* Dr. F. Batmanghelidj says that chronic cellular dehydration painfully and prematurely kills. Its initial outward manifestations have until now been labeled as "diseases of unknown origin".

Dr. Batmanghelidj says we need to drink ½ ounce of water each and every day for every pound we weigh. If you are significantly dehydrated, you should gradually work up to the correct amount of water because your kidneys may not be ready for the amount of water you actually need. If you are seriously overweight, you may not be able to drink such a large amount of water, because it might cause low sodium. The time-honored recommendation is 64 oz. per day.

Drinking more water is not a panacea. You may still need help from doctors and therapists if your blood pressure is very high. Some people have been able to stop taking pharmaceutical drugs for high blood pressure by controlling their intake of water and salt. It helps if you have a battery-operated blood pressure machine so that you can check your blood pressure frequently. You can take charge of things in your life.

When you drink caffeinated or alcoholic beverages in place of water, you are causing dehydration, which is associated with obesity, digestive problems, aches and pains, headaches, depression, allergies, elevated blood cholesterol and Alzheimer's disease. So, what you drink and what you don't drink can cause stress that distracts your body from healing.

44. Eleven Ways to Gain Weight Without Really Trying

By: Dr. Judith Giustini

1. PIGGING-0UT, HIGH CALORIE FAST FOODS: Excess calories get stored as fat.

2. SLIGHTLY OVEREATING, NIBBLING: When you eat 3,500 calories over your maintenance level, you gain one pound.

3. HYPOGLYCEMIA: Low blood sugar is an emergency for your brain. You will eat "anything" to fix it.

4. YO-YO DIETING: Lose weight, gain it again.

5. DIABETES: If your cells are sick, they won't want to take in more nutrients. Excess blood sugar gets stored as fat.

6. DEHYDRATION: Your brain uses energy from sugar and "hydroelectricity" from water. Thirst is mistaken for hunger.

7. SODA: Bubbly, tasty, caffeine and lots of empty calories.

8. COFFEE: Caffeine is addicting. Some coffee drinks contain as many as 700 empty calories.

9. DIET SODA: Sweet taste makes your body expect nutrients and stop burning stored calories. No food found induces hunger.

10. EMPTY CALORIES: Starvation in the midst of plenty

11. LACK OF EXERCISE: Walking burns 100 cal./mile.

45. Eliminate Empty Calories

By: Dr. Judith Giustini

Breakfast: Oops no time or maybe a donut & coffee

Coffee Break: Soda and chips

Lunch: Burger, Fries, Soda

      For kids: versions of same

Coffee Break: Coffee and candy bar

Dinner: Meat, potatoes and vegetable or could be pizza, burgers and soda or alcohol

Evening Snacks: Chips, sodas, beers, cookies, ice cream . . .

The empty calorie diet is a prescription for obesity, hypoglycemia, diabetes, heart trouble and chronic fatigue.

The original diet of mankind, going back to Adam and Eve, was plant based. Animal flesh as a food did not come in until after the flood of Noah's day.

You may be able to get along on a diet of empty calories "for a while", but if your body does not have the nutrients it needs to do its job, it will start breaking down.

Empty calorie foods are tasty and easy to get and eat, but if you eat them, your body will have to supply the enzymes and digesting fluids to process them, thus placing additional stress on your digestive system and many other systems.

Your body needs nutrients to keep your immune system running optimally. Viruses are all around, waiting to get you. Once you run your health into the ground, it is hard to get it back up and going. The nursing homes are welcoming new residents. You can eliminate empty calories.

46. Enzymes (from multiple research sources)

By: Dr. Judith Giustini

Enzymes are proteins that increase the rates of chemical reactions.

Enzymes from barley are used by yeast to ferment beer.Enzymes from papaya are used to tenderize meat.Enzymes are used to remove stains from your clothing.Penicillin and Aspirin work because of enzymes.Ptyalin and Amylase are saliva enzymes that break down foods.Lipase is a stomach enzyme that splits fats.Renin is a stomach enzyme that curdles milk.Pepsin is a stomach enzyme that helps digest proteins.

Enzymes facilitate metabolism to supply the needs of your cells. Your body's production of enzymes depends on the availability of the materials to make them and the health of your organs. If you have spent a long time on a diet of empty calories, you may not have enough ingredients and your organs may be too sick to produce your enzymes. You may need to take digestive enzyme tablets to help digest your food. Fresh raw fruits and vegetables contain enzymes to digest themselves, so they don't need to use your body's enzymes.

Digestive enzymes work in digestive *juices.* Dehydration will interfere with your digestion. According to Dr. F. Batmanghelidj in his book *Your Body's Many Cries for Water,* you need ½ ounce of water per day per pound you weigh, however, this may be unrealistic if you are very heavy. For many years, doctors have been recommending 8 - 8 oz. glasses of water per day, same as a major weight loss group.

47. Excess Body Weight

By: Dr. Judith Giustini

Conventional wisdom says that obesity is due to overeating. If you are a woman, you will burn about 2,000 calories per day. If you overeat by 100 calories per day, you will gain one pound every 35 days – that's at least 10 lbs. per year. If you are a man, you can consume about 2,500 calories per day before you start packing on the pounds.

All foods contain calories, but some foods are not good for you. This amazing body that (hopefully) still lets you walk around and breathe air, is a gift from Someone who loves you very much. If your car burns gasoline, you wouldn't fill the tank with diesel fuel, would you? You wouldn't let it run out of oil. Can you be as kind to your own body?

Obesity is fraught with emotional and physical dilemmas. You may be confused and afraid to try another weight loss program because of so many disappointments in the past. You need a simple plan.

In Chapter 8 of his book *Your Body's Many Cries for Water,* Dr. F. Batmanghelidj discusses the importance of consuming the appropriate amount of water for yourself if you are on a weight loss diet. Some people have lost their excess lbs. by just changing this one thing. Eliminate refined sugar and white flour. That could represent hundreds of calories per day.

Next, change to a plant-based diet. If you consume 1200 per day for a woman or 1,500 calories per day for a man, you will definitely lose weight and be taking good care of your body.

48. Exercise as a Cause of Stress that Can Interfere with Healing

By: Dr. Judith Giustini

Exercise is a complicated subject because there are so many forms of exercise, each person is of a different age and fitness level and everyone has different opportunities and inclinations to exercise.

Exercise in moderation is said to be good for you. It stimulates the release of feel-good hormones. It helps your heart and blood vessels and keeps your muscles toned up. If you are fit, you can get around easier and accomplish your tasks.

Conventional wisdom says that people who need to lose weight should decrease their intake of food and increase their amount of exercise. But exercise may not be advisable if you are obese or sick. You might have to work on your health first, and incorporate exercise into your schedule. very gradually.

"EWO" (Exercising While Obese) can be very stressful on your cardiovascular system, your hips and your knees. If you exercise while dehydrated, this can cause more problems.

If you are already feeling not-too-well about yourself, and you go to a gym and see many people who look better in spandex than you do, this can be humiliating and make you want to go and hide. Some of those thin people may have been pretty pudgy before they started their exercise program at the gym.

If exercise causes an emotional overwhelm that puts you into defense physiology, it can actually make you sick. The fight-or-flight mode is opposite to the healing mode.

49. Exhaustion: Your Ticket to the Nursing Home

By: Dr. Judith Giustini

Exhaustion happens to you as the result of stress. You can have stress from your lifestyle choices, your environment, your relationships, your conscious and your subconscious thoughts, feelings, beliefs and memories.

Your body can go along for a while, compensating for your eating and drinking things that are not good for you or failing to drink enough water. It can also deal with the stress of your negative thinking for a while, but eventually it will no longer be able to cope. System after system will become overwhelmed and break down. You may end taking multiple prescription drugs and not feeling better. Exhaustion depletes your immune system, making it difficult for your body to contend with viruses and germs.

Do you know how much water your body needs each day to do its job of keeping you alive? Dr. F. Batmanghelidj (watercure.com) says you need ½ ounce of water (plus 1 tsp. of sea salt per gallon) per day per pound you weigh. Just making that one lifestyle change can help you avoid obesity, diabetes, heart trouble, Parkinson's disease, Alzheimer's disease and more.

A high protein diet leads to "acidosis", which is a feature in gout, arthritis, and diabetes. You can learn to test the pH of your urine and know the meaning of the test results, so you can tailor your diet to be most beneficial to you.

To avoid Exhaustion, you may need to take charge of some unresolved subconscious negative feelings.

50. Fat Affects Everything

By: Dr. Judith Giustini

Right now, millions of people are suffering the effects of war, floods, earthquakes, financial crisis and diseases of all sorts. If you are sitting here with 50 to 200 lbs. of extra weight on your body, this can be almost as stressful as dealing with a calamity, but it goes on 24/7 and seems to have no resolution.

You are aware of your fat when you turn over in bed, walk across the room or walk across a street. You can't move fast; your heart pounds and you sweat. Maybe you are a candidate for hip or knee replacement. Maybe you ride the motorized vehicle in Walmart because you are in pain when you walk.

You are aware of your fat when the weather is warm, when you are in a small kitchen or bathroom. When you are sitting at the table, sitting in a booth or in a seat in an airplane.

You are aware of your fat when you shop for clothing. Maybe you shop for plus-size clothing online or on TV to save embarrassment or physical exertion.

Your fat is may have motivated you to go on a diet, and you quickly regained all the weight you lost. If you are going to become a normal weight person, you are going to have to make a lifestyle change. Maybe your fat can motivate you to take charge of things in your life.

Maybe you could take some time and create a list of the things in your life that fat is affecting and make a picture in your mind of how you choose things to be when you are a normal weight person. When you have a goal in your mind, the steps to getting there will present themselves. It's up you to you to set the goal and take the steps to get it done.

51. Fat People Are Sick

By: Dr. Judith Giustini

Fat people may not "look" sick. Maybe they look "healthy" or "robust", but they don't feel that way. Obesity has come to be the new normal. Plus sizes are in stores and on TV. Women can rent plus-size outfits and send them back. Many children are obese.

In my Weight Watcher's class, the speaker asked, "How did _you_ get fat?" and then she proceeded to tell about her own experiences of going out to pick up a pizza for the family, and eating a whole pizza on the way home, nibbling a bag of candy bars, while driving around in her car, etc.

The foods that make you fat are usually "empty calorie" foods. They taste great going down, but they do not supply essential vitamins, minerals or fiber. Soda and other beverages do not take the place of water. Malnutrition and dehydration are the pathway to diabetes, high blood pressure and chronic degenerative disease.

Obesity is only the most obvious symptom of a whole underlying problem of illness, where every little cell in your body is not playing with a full deck. As more and more cells lose the game, your organ systems start to fail and there are limited resources in your body to repair them. New symptoms join old symptoms: fibromyalgia, chronic fatigue, incontinence, arthritis, etc.

If you decide to stop allowing fat to make you sick, you should make an assessment of where you are starting out from What is your weight, your blood pressure, your saliva pH, your urine pH, the results of your 5-hour glucose tolerance test, your blood cholesterol, etc. You need to know if unresolved subconscious negative feelings are affecting you. You may need help to get you over this illness of obesity. There is no shame in accepting help, but you have to consider the source and the intent.

52. Fat People DO Car

By: Dr. Judith Giustini

Two normal weight people were having a conversation in Walmart, when a morbidly obese person rode by on a motorized shopping vehicle. The man, on seeing this, said. "Fat people just don't care." Where did he get his information? Has he spoken to any fat people lately?

If you are a fat person, your obesity may be causing you to be discriminated against in the workplace, maybe overlooked for promotions or maybe not hired in the first place. If you are looking for love on a dating site, you may be a very nice person, but some people draw the line at fatties, so forget about the coffee date.

If you are a fat person, your fat MAKES you care. It's on your mind 24/7, interfering with your activities of daily living, your choice of jobs, your social life, your shopping, your cooking, your housekeeping, you're driving, etc. Your fat is like a person that goes around with you all the time, has to be considered in every situation, and sometimes it gets you to eat and drink all the wrong things.

If you are tired of being a subject for ridicule by strangers in Walmart, you are going to have to find out what is causing your fat. Obesity is a very complicated subject. It has to do with what you eat drink and breathe and how you exercise, rest, and think. Part of a weight loss program is mathematics. If you burn more calories than you take in, you will lose weight.

Your lifestyle choices are motivated by deep seated programming in your subconscious mind. You may need the help of a weight loss group and a mind-body therapist so you can take charge of things in your life.

53. What You Eat as a Cause of Stress

that Interferes with Healing

By: Dr. Judith Giustini

Your choices of what you eat are dictated by complex influences that go deep into your subconscious belief system.

Your food choices are also influenced by information you observe in TV advertising of foods that look yummy, even though they might be very high in calories and very low in nutrients.

Some foods were not meant to be eaten. These are things such as shellfish and pork. They are listed in Chapter 11 of the book of Leviticus in The Bible. Many people still eat margarine, which is chemically one molecule away from plastic. Flies and rats won't eat it, so why should we?

Poor choices of what you eat and drink can cause a problem in your acid-alkaline balance that causes interference in your body's ability to heal itself. A diet that is too high in protein causes an acid condition in your blood that interferes with your red blood cells being able to transport oxygen, and this can lead to a heart attack. This same chemistry results in osteoporosis, diabetes, gout and arthritis.

You only have so many days to live on this planet. The foods you choose to eat can help these days to be comfortable or uncomfortable. If your acid-alkaline balance is causing a life and death emergency in your body, this may interfere with your body's being able to resist a viral infection.

54. Foods Forbidden in the Bible

By: Dr. Judith Giustini

In Leviticus Ch. 11, God spoke directly with Moses and Aaron about the foods His people could eat and should avoid.

He said you may eat every creature that splits the hoof and chews the cud.

Some animals He said not to eat are: the camel, the rock badger, the hare, and the pig. About pigs, He said that you must not eat any of their flesh or touch their dead body because they are unclean for you.

He said you can eat everything from the waters that has fins and scales. (This excludest shellfish and catfish.)

Among the flying creatures, you are not to eat are the eagle, the osprey, the vulture, the raven, the ostrich, the owl, the gull, the swan, the pelican and the bat.

I Timothy 4:1-4 would seem to indicate that all foods are okay to eat. However, careful reading of I Timothy 4:3 shows that this is referring to *"foods which God created to be partaken of"*. Leviticus Ch. 11 tells you what they are and what they are not. Moses and Aaron and The Israelites had bodies like our own. Eating the wrong foods will make you sick.

You can look up Leviticus Ch. 11 to get the full story.

55. Fruits & Vegetables & Your Weight Loss Diet

By: Dr. Judith Giustini

If you are having trouble with your weight, you might also have diabetes, arthritis, gallstones, osteoporosis, kidney, liver or heart disease, all of which are very common in overweight people. All of these conditions are associated with what you eat and drink. This is bad in one way, because you have to acknowledge your own part in causing the problem, but good in another way, because this means that you have the power to change what you have been doing to cause it.

If you are trying to lose weight, you need to restrict your calories to 1,200 for a woman and 1,500 calories for a man. Fruits and vegetables are low in calories (Ch. 171) and you can consume moderate portions of them without going over your calorie limit. (Ch. 164. Super Soup, 165. Super Shakes) They also help to keep you alkaline, which is a good state for your general health and for facilitating weight loss. You can learn to monitor your urinary pH (Ch. 123.).

If you choose a plant-based diet, you may opt to have eggs and milk in moderation. Beans and white and sweet potatoes are good. You have to count the calories (Ch. 171.)

A major contributor to obesity is dehydration. In Dr. F. Batmanghelidj's book *You're Not Sick, You're Thirsty!* he tells you the physiological causes of many "conditions of unknown origin" that are called diseases, but they are actually the body's way of coping with dehydration. It is very difficult to re-train your habits to accommodate drinking the water you need. It is important to discipline yourself.

56. The Yo-Yo Weight Syndrome

By: Dr. Judith Giustini

How much do you weigh now? What is your goal weight?

If you are obese, you know how that makes you feel, maybe not so happy with yourself, despite the fact that you have a lot of pudgy folks for company these days.

Maybe you have tried different diets with various degrees of success, but something always happens, and your weight creeps up again? Too bad about all those new thinner-person clothes you just bought.

If you are obese, that means you have consumed too many calories, and your body has stored them as fat. There is a formula for losing weight, which is 1,200 calories per day for a woman and 1,500 calories per day for a man. On this program, you will lose about 2 lbs. per week (maybe more right at first if you are starting out from very heavy), but you have to STICK TO IT 24/7, week in and week out.

There are calories and there are calories. Some calories are found in nutritious foods that nourish you and help you become or stay healthy, and some calories are "empty calories", such as those found in products containing white flour and sugar. Maybe you can develop "Calorie Consciousness" (Ch. 162.), and then graduate to "Nutritional Awareness" (Ch. 163.). Obesity is terrible for your health, happiness. and success. Maybe you went on a diet before, and you lost some weight, but it came right back when you returned to your old diet. You can choose to Divorce Your Old Diet (Ch. 41.) and use this opportunity to take charge of things in your life. You may need professional help.

57. How Does Childhood Obesity Lead to Adult Obesity?

By: Dr. Judith Giustini

People who are obese as children are more likely to be obese as adults because more fat cells are formed during infancy and early childhood. People obese as children may have five times more fat cells than people of normal weight.

The number of fat cells cannot be reduced, so weight can be lost only by markedly decreasing the fat in each cell. This fact may limit how much weight can be lost and make maintaining a normal weight more difficult.

Fat children are fat for the same reasons that fat adults are fat. Fat children can have diabetes and high blood pressure just the same as adults who are fat.

Gone are the days when schoolchildren used to eat a nutritious breakfast at home and homemade sandwich and fruit for lunch. Some children eat breakfast, lunch and dinner at fast food places. The convenience store next to the school yard is replete with candy, soda and chips. It is easy to become addicted to this kind of diet and become a fat person for life.

If your schoolchild is obese, wouldn't it be nice if they could attend an educational program about the nutritional content of foods and what diet they need to follow to help themselves be healthy, and this will contribute to their happiness and success. Maybe they could have a cooking class and a dining table, so they could put the information they are learning into practice. They might find out they like culinary arts as a career or just learn to help themselves and their families to live better.

58. How Does Dehydration Cause Excess Weight?

By: Dr. Judith Giustini

If you mistake thirst for hunger, you might tend to eat food instead of drinking water. You will continue to be dehydrated and you will not have the water your body needs as an energy source for the physiological reactions your body needs to perform.

Dr. Batmanghelidj (watercure.com) says that if you drink enough water, you don't need to count calories. Your taste buds and your satiety mechanism will do the work. Drink water before eating food and give it time to override your perception of hunger.

The regular intake of water will keep your body in fat-breaking mode until you take your next sugary or starchy food. They encourage insulin-induced fat storage and "hypoglycemic panics" that force you to eat more of the same.

Dr. Batmanghelidj said that it is not the fat content of your diet that causes heart disease. It is chronic unintentional dehydration – and its associated mineral deficiencies that is the primary cause of heart problems.

When your daily diet does not include adequate water, you do not properly absorb the minerals in your food. This is when your body becomes acidic, and your acidic blood eats into the delicate arterial membranes. Dark yellow or orange urine means an acidic body, indicating of the onset of heart disease. You are the only person who can drink your water.

59. How Many Calories are in Beverages?

By: Dr. Judith Giustini

A well-known chain of donut restaurants has an extensive menu of beverages. The calorie content ranges from zero calories in a plain coffee to 799 calories in a medium frozen coffee ice cream drink. Soda sweetened with sugar or corn syrup is about 150 calories per 12 ounces. A medium vanilla shake at a fast-food place is 550 calories.

You do not have to wonder how many calories are in what beverage because you can go online and find out from the website of the company that is serving the beverage or go to websites that list the calorie content of beverages.

Alcoholic beverages can be a real problem when you are trying to lose weight. 1 ounce of liquor contains 80-90 calories. 12 oz. of 8% beer contains 150 calories and wines contain about 200 calories per serving. Some folks cut back on good food, so they can drink alcohol and not gain weight.

As soon as alcohol is consumed, it is used as energy, while the calories from food may be stored as fat. Alcohol tends to stimulate your appetite and reduce your self-control. The extra calories from the alcohol and the extra food you are likely to eat can ruin several days of hard work staying on your diet.

Plan ahead to be sure you are not drinking your way to overconsuming calories and stopping your body from losing weight. Water is your best choice. Diet soda contains an artificial sweetener that is getting some bad reviews. The artificial sweet taste makes your body think food is going to be there and it causes you to eat.

60. How Many Calories Are in Foods?

By: Dr. Judith Giustini

A few years ago, you had to go to a bookstore and get a book to find out how many calories there are in foods. These days, you can Google "calories in natural foods" or "calories in fast-foods" or "calories in Chinese foods" or calories according to the name of the restaurant chain or donut house. (Ch. 169)

Using this information, you can know ahead of time about what will go on your plate and in your beverage cup each day.

At one dairy place, a vanilla soft serve cone is 140 calories, a medium chocolate shake is 760 calories, hamburgers are 290 – 1,180 calories, French fries are 380 calories per medium serving and onion rings are 470 calories.

At a burger place, hamburgers and chicken sandwiches contain 260-860 calories. Medium French fries are 380 calories, an egg muffin sandwich is 300 calories and deluxe breakfast is 1,220 calories. Some chain restaurants have several items on their menus that would fit in with a weight loss diet. If you are doing Defensive Dining (Ch. 37.), you will study their menu ahead of time, so you know what you are going to order when you get there.

One restaurant's onion ring are 1,289 calories and their fish and chips are 1,689 calories. They do have some items on their menu that would fit in with your weight loss diet, but their customers and their serving people all seem to be heavy.

One restaurant offers French bread with maple butter syrup and bacon or ham. It is 2,780 calories. First place winner.

61. How Much Food Do You Need to Eat to Feel Satisfied?

By: Dr. Judith Giustini

A pudgy woman in her 60's took insulin for her diabetes. For work, she took care of children in her home – usually one child at a time. She liked to work from home so that she would be near her kitchen because she had a strong attachment to food, going back to her childhood when she often went to bed hungry. She said she had tried to lose weight, but she needed a to feel a certain degree of fullness in her stomach to feel satisfied, so she remained fat.

A few years ago, there were "fat shows" on TV. On these shows, morbidly obese people would go to a camp, where they would eat less and exercise more. Some of the people complained about the size of food portions, which were actually quite large.

Some people would not feel satisfied on a diet that only allows small portions, but foods vary widely in the number of calories they contain. One cup of green beans is about 30 calories and one cup of ice cream is about 300 calories.

In the program of a very successful weight loss group, most vegetables are unlimited, so you don't have to count the calories and you can eat as much as you want. You can learn some low-calorie toppings for your vegetables to make them seem tasty to you. Vegetables are full of nutrients in a highly absorbable form. You can use them as an ingredient in Super Soup (Ch. 164.) and Super Shakes (Ch. 165.).

If you have a lot of weight to lose, you may be saving your life with this diet. Take time to figure out what works for you.

62. How Much Protein Do You Need?

By: Dr. Judith Giustini

Protein is important. Protein is a major component of your 75 trillion cells. Proteins are necessary for growth and healing of tissues. Your DNA and your hair are made of protein.

The Recommended Daily Allowance for protein is about 46-56 grams of protein per day, depending on age, sex and health condition. 4 oz. of beef contains 22 grams of protein, 190 calories.4 oz. of chicken contains 18 grams of protein, 125 calories4 oz. cottage cheese contains 20 grams of protein, 100 calories.1 med. egg contains 6 grams of protein, 75 calories. Vegetables, beans and grains contain protein.

After metabolism, proteins from plant sources leave a weak acid residue that can be eliminated through your lungs. Proteins from animal sources leave a strong acid that needs to be neutralized before it can pass through your kidneys. The organic sodium from fruits and vegetables is used to neutralize this strong acid. If organic sodium is not available, your body will take calcium from your teeth and bones to neutralize it.

After a while on excessive protein, there is a point at which no amount of fruits and vegetables will supply enough minerals to neutralize the acid. Your body will become exhausted, and you may have a heart attack, arthritis, osteoporosis, or diabetes, but you might not realize you caused it with your food choices. Excess protein intake will show up in your urine pH. You can learn to monitor your urine pH and know what the results mean. (Ch. 63. How's Your Urine pH?, Ch. 127. What is Your Alkaline Reserve?)

63. How's Your Urine pH?

By: Dr. Judith Giustini

When you test your first morning urine with yellow pH paper, the paper will either remain yellow, turn green or turn blue. Yellow is 5.5 (Acid), blue is 8.0 (Alkaline) greens are in-between. The pH of your urine reflects the pH of the foods you have been consuming recently.

When you are born and when you die, the pH of your urine is 8.0. There is an obvious difference between a newborn baby and a dead person. The baby's urine is alkaline because it has consumed alkaline minerals from its mother's diet and stores of alkalinity, such as the calcium from her teeth and bones.

The alkalinity of the dying person is caused by the body's response to excess acid that has been neutralized by the body's production of ammonia, which is very alkaline.

If you consume a diet that is mostly fruits and vegetables, your urine test strip will be greenish. If you consume a diet that is mostly animal proteins and grains, your urine test strip might be yellow, which shows it is not too overwhelmed with dietary stress to be able to heal. When you get into the emergency mode due to excess of acid-ash foods the blue on your test strip is a sign that you are in the "survival" mode, not in the healing mode.

Your body was designed to operate optimally in a slightly alkaline state due to consumption of fruits and vegetables. This is also the pH that is most conducive to keeping you at your optimal weight. Excess consumption of acid-ash (high protein) foods makes your blood less capable of transporting oxygen to the cells all over your body, including your heart.

64. Hunger, Appetite and Food Cravings

By: Dr. Judith Giustini

From Wikipedia:

HUNGER: The physical sensation of desiring food because of being unable to eat sufficient food to meet nutritional needs. Wars and adverse weather conditions have caused hunger. High food prices contribute to hunger.

APPETITE: The desire to eat food, felt as hunger. Regulates energy intake for metabolic needs through interplay between digestive tract, adipose tissue and brain.

FOOD CRAVING: An intense desire to consume a specific food like chocolate. May be associated with low levels of feel-good brain chemicals. Food can become an addiction, like alcohol.

What you choose to eat is dictated by your programming, your body image, your blood sugar, your nutrient needs and maybe by what your mother ate when she was pregnant to you.

If you consume 500 calories per day fewer than it takes to maintain your weight for 7 days, you will lose one pound.

You might experience hunger when your blood sugar is low or when you are dehydrated. It will help you to have frequent small meals of natural foods and drink at least64 oz. of water per day.

If you are in a General Rundown Condition due to long-term nutritional deficiencies, dehydration and emotional stress, it is going to take WORK for you to get well, if you still can.

65. If Fat is the Problem, what is the Solution?

By: Dr. Judith Giustini

If you are fat, you are not alone. About 40% of U.S. adults and 30% of U.S. children are obese. Fat is a terrible problem to fat people. If you are fat and you hate what fat is doing to your work life, your social life and your love life, you may have tried various fad diets unsuccessfully. Trying one more thing that also might not work might be daunting, considering the current state of your hopes.

If you choose to become a normal-weight person, you are embarking on a journey that will take you the rest of your life, sometimes going uphill. You will be doing battle with the programming of your subconscious belief system and your time-honored habits of what you eat, drink, and think. You may be chronically dehydrated. Maybe you have PTSD.

If you are frustrated with your fat, you may have many unresolved subconscious negative feelings dating back to whenever, and you may have a lot of negative feelings towards ourself for being in this condition. If you are a person who eats when you are upset, being upset about your obesity might send you to the cookie department and you will have failed to consume fewer calories than you burn, and you will have to start over again tomorrow.

You can become a normal-weight person if you commit to a plant-based diet that is low in calories and high in nutrients and water. You can eat plenty of food on this diet, only not the same foods that made you fat. (Ch. 162., 163., 165.) That is the solution. You will have to take charge of things in your life for the long haul. Hopefully, this book can be your little friend, and hold your hand along the way.

66. Just Eat Less

By: Dr. Judith Giustini

What you eat and how much you eat are dictated by many complicated factors. You might be in a habit of eating a breakfast of juice, pancakes with butter and syrup, eggs, ham or bacon and coffee with cream and sugar. This meal can be 1,000 calories or more. A burger, fries and soda for lunch can be another 1,000 calories. A dinner of steak and potatoes or pizza with beverages can be another 1,000 calories. What about the calories in your snacks throughout the day and evening? If you are a man whose body burns 2,500 calories per day or a woman who burns 2,000 calories per day, it is easy to consume more calories than you burn.

One evening, there were 950 lbs. of ladies sitting in 3 chairs in for a seminar about nutrition. One of the ladies weighed about 350 lbs. She had diabetes and she was experiencing deteriorating vision, leg cramps when walking, and numbness and tingling in her fingers and toes. She quit drinking soda and high calorie coffee drinks for 3 months she and lost 50 lbs.

If you consume 500 calories per day fewer than you burn for one week, you will lose 1 lb. This sounds simple, but it is not easy because of all your habits and your social situation. For you to get into your lifetime lifestyle change, you may have to work on many large and small lifestyle choices and the stress of your negative thoughts, feelings beliefs and memories. You may have to reconsider the with whom, where, what, why, when and how of everything you eat drink and think.

A positive attitude is useful in this situation.

67. And Exercise More

By: Dr. Judith Giustini

Walking one mile for a person of "normal" weight burns about 100 calories. The more you weigh, the more calories it takes to move the mass over the distance. A heavy woman in our little town began walking many miles per day, carrying her phone and music in a backpack. After a while, people who saw her walking every day began to recognize that she was losing weight. Eventually, she became noticeably slim.

A man used to weigh 250 lbs. when he played minor league football. He hurt his knee and had to have 4 surgeries. He spent 2 years resting his leg and receiving therapy. By the time he was up and around, he weighed 400 lbs. He was able to get a job as a front door security person at electronics store. He was losing weight on a diet, but exercise was not an option.

A woman who fell and hurt her right knee walking to grade school reinjured the same knee a couple of times in falls. She reinjured her right knee again in a workplace injury and she had trouble just walking across the parking lot to her office. Staying home on workmen's compensation and following her total knee replacement, she turned to macaroni salad and cookies to calm her anxiety and she gained 100 lbs.

A woman who weighed about 250 lbs. decided to enroll in a gym. When she was in classes next to people who weighed 100 lbs. less than she did, she felt out of place. Also, she was unable to perform most of the exercises. She opted for a treadmill in her home and she was diligent about using it, meanwhile taking charge of the calories in her diet and she lost 100 lbs.

68. Starvation in the Midst of Plenty

By: Dr. Judith Giustini

Back in the day, people ate most of their meals at home. Whole foods grown on healthy soils . . . But today, we are so advanced. We have refined foods and drive-through restaurants. Donut, anybody?

Your body was designed to operate with certain amounts of proteins, fats, carbohydrates, vitamins, minerals and water. Too bad they don't teach this in 7th grade. It is thought that in a few years, 50% of the people will be obese. Because they have been living on a Typical American Diet, they are malnourished and maybe dehydrated. But their old diet is so "comfortable". Being heavy, they can consume more calories without gaining more weight. Their social life is based on dining with friends and family.

If you are not feeling well, nobody is going to come along and spoon feed you the nutritional information you need to know. Fortunately, there is a plethora of information online. You just have to ask. If you need to lose weight, you will need to stick to a diet of 1,200 calories per day if you are a woman and 1,500 calories per day if you are a man. (Ch. 163. The Super Shakes Plan and 164. Implementing the Super Shakes Plan).

At first, you might feel "greedy" for your Super Shakes. This is because your body has been so starving, and it wants to grab all the nutrients it can. This will subside after a while, and it will be easier to stay within your calorie allowance. Maybe you will be motivated to move on from Calorie Consciousness to Nutritional Awareness.

69. Minerals are Essential for Your Health

By: Dr. Judith Giustini

Recently, many articles have been published saying that there is no clear benefit to multivitamin and mineral products, their use is not justified, and they should be avoided. Your best source of vitamins and minerals is natural foods. Check it out.

Calcium, found in dairy products, green leafy vegetables and certain algae products. Some calcium products contain a substance from rocks that is not soluble in your body Calciumis necessary for growth and maintenance of teeth and bones.

Copper, found in cooked oysters, cashew nuts and veal liver, Is essential for absorption of iron. Deficiency results in anemia.

Iodine, found in baked potatoes with peel, iodized salt and cooked beans, is necessary for proper thyroid function.

Iron, found in spinach, chard, pumpkin seeds and dark chocolate, is used to transport oxygen to all parts of the body.

Magnesium, found in spinach, squash seeds, fish and dark chocolate, is necessary for muscle and nerve function.

Manganese, found in hazelnuts, and whole wheat bread, is necessary for enzyme function and wound healing.

Phosphorous, found in pumpkin seeds, yogurt and salmon, is necessary for making energy and strong bones and teeth.

Potassium, found in baked potato, beans and yogurt, is necessary to maintain fluid and electrolyte balance.

Sodium, found in table salt and foods to which it is added, Is necessary for proper blood pressure and nerve signaling.

Selenium, found in Brazil nuts, tuna, beef and lamb, is necessary for proper function of the thyroid gland.

Zinc, found in oysters, beef, lamb and pumpkin seeds, is necessary for sense of smell, immune system. See if you can find sea salt that contains natural minerals

70. Nutrition is Involved in Six of the Ten
Leading Causes of Death in the United States

By: Dr. Judith Giustini

The ten leading causes of death in the U.S. are: heart disease, cancer, injuries from accidents, lung disease, stroke, Alzheimer's disease, diabetes, influenza, kidney disease and suicide. Obesity is a predisposing factor in at least six of them.

Every one of your trillions of cells needs certain nutrients to function optimally. You feel uncomfortable when you are hungry, so you go ahead and eat something to assuage your hunger. What you choose to eat may taste good and fill you up, even though it is not the not be the best thing for your health. You, the person walking around and breathing air had a choice of what was on your dinner plate, but your trillions of little cell "people" don't have a choice. They can only pick and choose from whatever you put on the menu.

If your cells are starving, your organ systems will begin to break down. Which illness develops, when and how, will depend on which cells are affected by your nutritional choices, plus the effects of many other stressors.

Your cells need the nutrients from whole foods. Fragmented foods do not have the same nutritional value. A plant-based diet of 80% fruits and vegetables, and 20% everything else, has been recommended by the most astute authorities innutrition.

Water is said to be the most essential nutrient. In his book *Your Body's Manu Cries for Water*, Dr. F. Batmanghelidj says that many illnesses labeled as "diseases of unknown origin" are actually the physiological effects of dehydration.

71. Obesity

By: Dr. Judith Giustini

Around the world, more than 50 million adults and children per year die of starvation. 80% of malnourished children live in countries that produce food surpluses. Wars lead to homelessness and refugee camps. Weather events displace many people. Heart disease is the leading cause of death in the US, claiming the lives of about 800,000 persons annually.

At the same time as the famines are going on and people are dying of starvation, childhood obesity in the U.S. has reached epidemic proportions and it is spreading around in the developed and developing world. Obesity of children and adults is one of the leading preventable causes of death worldwide. In the United States, about 300,000 people die of obesity each year and it is a factor in many co-morbities

Obesity doubles or triples your risk of premature death. Moderate obesity reduces life expectancy by six to seven years. Severe obesity reduces life expectancy by about ten years. Obese people tend to have more kidney disease, cardiovascular disease, Type 2 diabetes, cancer, strokes, high blood pressure, high cholesterol and osteoarthritis. That's six out of ten of the leading causes of death.

2/3 of US adults are and 1/3 of children are obese. It would seem that we would get accustomed to looking at them and nothing would seem amiss. But no. Even if you are obese, you can still look at another obese person and feel that something is wrong with this picture.

Aside from being life-threatening, obesity is annoying to obese people. It interferes with your functions of daily living, and it takes a serious toll on your health, happiness, and success.

72. Obesity, The Law of Attraction and The Law of Cause & Effect

By: Dr. Judith Giustini

According to <u>The Law of Cause & Effect</u>, if you consume more calories than you burn, you will gain weight. Why you consume more calories than you burn is a very complicated matter that involves your belief system, your programming, your memories and the subconscious feelings that are associated with them.

According to <u>The Law of Attraction</u>, you attract your experiences and relationships that resonate with the vibrations of the feelings buried alive in your subconscious mind. Maybe, with your conscious mind (10% of thinking), you choose to be a normal-weight person, but some negative feelings in your subconscious mind are very powerful attractors of obesity. Certain feelings tend to attract the symptom pattern identified as "Fat" and other feelings attract you to "Over-Eating". If merely eating less and exercising more has not been working out for you, you might benefit from some Mind-Body Therapy sessions, so you can find out the feelings you need to let go of and the feelings you need to replace them with.

According to Dr. F. Batmanghelidj in his book *Obesity, Cancer & Depression,* chronic cellular dehydration is a major cause of obesity. Many of his patients lost their extra lbs. merely by increasing their consumption of water to the right amount for themselves, which he says is ½ oz. per day for every pound you weigh, plus 1 tsp. of sea salt, per gallon of water. If you are quite heavy, this could be a lot of water. Maybe excessive? Maybe try 64 oz. per day as recommended by international weight loss group?

73. Obesity and "Betrayed"

By: Dr. Judith Giustini

Wikipedia defines BETRAYAL as "the breaking or violating of a presumptive contract, trust or confidence that produces moral and psychological conflict within a relationship".

Each obese person has a complicated background and many reasons for the negative feelings that are buried alive in their subconscious mind. In her book *Feelings Buried Alive Never Die,* Karol K. Truman provides an extensive list of illnesses and several feelings that may predispose a person to have this illness. For example, some feelings that may lead to the symptom pattern of *Fat* are listed as: "Feel a need for protection, Resistance to forgiving, and Hidden anger". She lists the feelings behind *Obesity* as: "Using food as a substitute for affection, Inability to admit to self and others what you really desire, Inability to express true feelings, seeking love, Protecting the body, trying to fulfill the self, and Stuffed feelings".

In Mind-Body Therapy, we are able to identify the underlying motivation and the feeling that is connected with it and the events or situations that are inciting it, possibly going back to their childhood. One feeling that has often been predisposing or causal has been "Betrayal". Maybe it's about something that happened long ago, and it's really "old news" by now. If t the person can Forgive their negative feelings about this, it will be one less thing to keep them running to the cookie jar. Forgiveness is "Winning by letting go", and the patient will be on a journey from Confusion to Self-Knowledge

If you let go of the negative feelings that are ending you up in the feeling of "Betrayed", you will have started on a journey that takes you from Confusion to Self-Awareness, and taking charge of things in your life.

74. Obesity as a Moneymaking Opportunity

By: Dr. Judith Giustini

The greater the number of obese people, the more opportunities there are for businesses to provide needed supplies and services:

Fitness Clubs
Home Weight Lifting Equipment
Aerobic Exercise Equipment
Sweat Pants and other Fitness/Workout Wear
Store for Used Gym Equipment
Exercise Shows on TV
Exercise DVD's - Zoomba, Beach Body, many others.
Weight_Watchers, Jenny Craig, Nutri-System
Clothing for Big People
"Fat Farms", Summer Weight Loss Camps
Diet Pills
Blood Sugar Testing Devices for Diabetics, Needles, etc.
Medical Doctors, Hospitals, Hip and Knee Replacements
Nutritionists
Counselors
Physical Therapists, Chiropractors
Nursing Homes
Therapy Facilities for Post-Hip and Knee Replacement Patients
Diabetes Drugs
High Blood Pressure Drugs
Refitting of Airline Cabins with Wider Seats
Wide-Load Office Chairs
Renovation of Office Areas to Make Room for Obese Employees
Pickup Trucks Instead of Cars for Obese Employees
Bigger Toilets for Obese People
    . . . and many more ways to make a buck on the pandemic of obesity.

75. Obesity is a Symptom

By: Dr. Judith Giustini

If you go in a supermarket in the U.S. today, you will observe numerous obese people pushing shopping baskets filled with empty-calorie foods and many bottles of soda.

You may see a morbidly obese person riding on a motorized vehicle because their hips, knees and low backs are not able to take the strain of walking around in such a large space.

Many people judge obese people, saying it is their own fault they are fat. But really, obesity is a symptom that has many causes, such as early programming of lifestyle choices (habits) through modeling by adults and what's available to eat and drink where you are when you get hungry.

You may not know how many calories you can consume per day without gaining weight, so the calorie content printed on food labels does not mean anything to you. You may have hypoglycemia, which causes you to reach for sugary snacks when your blood sugar gets low.

You may have unresolved negative feelings buried in your subconscious mind that keep running 24/7, causing you to be upset and nibbling on cookies to assuage your feelings of guilt, remorse, regret, etc.

According to Dr. F. Batmanghelidj in his book *Your Body's Many Cries for Water*, chronic cellular dehydration is a major cause of obesity. One woman reported that she weighed 35 lb.; less a couple of years earlier, when she was drinking 64 oz. of water per day and her low back, that was now in screaming pain, did not hurt when she was drinking enough water.

76. Obesity Increasing Among U.S. Preschoolers

By: Dr. Judith Giustini

From various sources:

15 to 30 percent of U.S. children 2 to 5 years of age are overweight. Studies have shown that obesity is more prevalent amongst certain ethnic groups and less prevalent in others.

Experts blame the prevalence of junk food marketed to children, too much TV and the decline in the number of families who sit down together to eat.

Some children drink 1-2 liters of soda per day. This can be about 600 – 1,200 empty calories per day, not including food. Soda is dehydrating. Caffeine is addicting. Water is the best beverage for those trying to lose weight. Some people have achieved a normal weight just by drinking the right amount of water for themselves every day.

By the time these obese children are in junior high school, many of them will have high triglycerides, high blood sugar, high blood pressure and a big waistline, and they will likely become obese adults.

77. "U.S. Life Expectancy May Drop Due to Obesity"

Report projects startling decline in longevity within next 50 years

By: Dr. Judith Giustini

An Associated Press article from Chicago, dated March 16, 2005said that U.S. life expectancy is expected to fall dramatically in coming years due to obesity.

It is predicted that the average lifespan of 77.6 years will be shortened by at least two to five years. That is more than the impact of cancer or heart disease. Some say this could inadvertently help "save" Social Security.

Two-thirds of U.S. adults are overweight or obese, as are one-third of U.S. children. Children as young as 4 years old are developing Type 2 diabetes. By the time they are in their teens, they may be experiencing the life-threatening complications of kidney disease, heart attack or stroke that only used to affect diabetics in their late 50's or 60's.

78. Prescription Medications for Weight Loss

By: Dr. Judith Giustini

Orlistat (from drugs.com) blocks some of the fat you eat, keeping it from being absorbed into your body. <u>Side-effects:</u> interferes with absorption of vitamins A, D, E and K, blood in urine, kidney problems, swelling in feet and ankles. Signs the medicine is working properly: oily or fatty stools, oily spotting in undergarments, gas and oily discharge, loose stools, inability to control bowel movements . . .

Sibutramine (from drugs.com) This drug was associated with cardiovascular events and strokes. It was taken off the market in several countries, including the United States.

Phentermine (from drugs.com) is a stimulant similar to an amphetamine. It acts as an appetite suppressant by affecting the central nervous system. <u>Side-effects:</u> feeling short of breath, even with mild exertion, chest pain, feeling like you might pass out, confusion, dangerously high B.P.

Benzphetamine (from drugs.com) is an "anorectic". It is recommended for use for only a few weeks. <u>Adverse Reactions:</u> Palpitation, rapid heartbeat, dizziness, nausea, diarrhea . . . Abuse may result in dependence and severe social dysfunction.

Diethylpropion (from WebMD) This drug is recommended for short term use by persons who are significantly overweight unable to lose weight on diet and exercise. It is an appetite suppressant. <u>Side-effects:</u> dizziness, insomnia, nausea, vomiting, diarrhea or constipation, high blood pressure.

Mazindol (from drugs.com). Removed from market.

Phendimetrazine (from drugs.com). Anorectic similar to amphetamines. Increases heart rate and blood pressure and decreases your <u>Side effects:</u> shortness of breath, swelling in ankles and feet, high blood pressure, impotence.

79. How to Reduce the High Cost of Health Care

By: Dr. Judith Giustini

Illness is expensive. The cost is more than just your co-pays or the payroll you are missing out on. Illness makes you upset and the stress of worrying about yourself can lead to further illness. Your illness is a drain on your family members if they need to help you or take over some of your duties, when they are already stressed from worrying about you.

What would happen if people seldom got sick? Think of the effect on our whole economy! This is not an unrealistic proposition if people would merely stop doing things that cause illness.

When you are sick or if you have a chronic degenerative disease, you may feel that you are a victim in a great conspiracy against your life. But what if you are the perpetrator of the scheme?

You may have to make changes what you eat, drink and breathe and how you exercise, rest and *THINK*.

Choose an alkaline diet. High protein foods and soda cause your system to be acid, resulting in illness. Adequately hydrate yourself. Dehydration is a factor in high blood pressure, obesity, Alzheimer's disease and more. Eliminate tobacco and bad drugs. Change your toxic thoughts. Learn what they are through Mind-Body Therapy.

If people are well, this is going to affect the profits of those in the hospital, nursing home, insurance and fast-food industries.

80. Should You Take Nutritional Supplements?

By: Dr. Judith Giustini

If you Google "Vitamins Unnecessary", you will find at least eleven articles on this subject, dating back several years. One article is called "The Multi-Vitamin Fallacy." Another says that American's "waste" $28 billion per year on vitamin supplements. Another says that taking vitamins is linked to higher a risk of death in older women.

The idea of some people about multi-vitamins is "might help, couldn't hurt". But what if your cells are already toxic and impaired? Maybe a big dose of synthetic compounds made in factories will give your little cells too big a job to do of detoxing these chemicals.

Your digestive system requires a lot of water to do its job. If you are dehydrated. and you consume something that needs to be denatured, this will increase the demand for water, and if it is not available, this will escalate the seriousness of your toxicity problem.

One reason you might consider taking multi-vitamin products is because you are feeling tired and rundown. There are many reasons for Exhaustion. Maybe you have PTSD due to adverse childhood experiences or mental-whiplash events. The stress of unresolved subconscious negative feelings can keep plaguing you minute to minute, day to day and you won't know why you feel so sick and tired.

If you are into Super Shakes (Ch. 163.) you might choose to add Spirulina, powdered kale, powdered hemp seeds, etc.

81. Signs of Mineral Deficiency

By: Dr. Judith Giustini

82

Flabby skin, weak muscles, osteoporosis, poor digestion, lethargy, abnormal heart rhythms, joint pain, lowered immunity, anemia, retardation in children, poor nutrient absorption, slow wound healing, weak bones and teeth, irritability, high blood pressure and loss of sense of smell are some effects of the deficiency of various minerals.

Minerals are essential for many complicated chemical reactions and functions throughout your body all the time. When minerals are not available in your diet and your body needs them for important purposes, such as keeping you alive, it will fetch them from your bones and other places where they are stored. When you have an injury, healing will be slow if your body doesn't have the minerals it needs to do the job

Some people who are deficient in essential minerals tend to eat more and more low nutrient foods to get the minerals their body needs for their chemical reactions. Empty calorie foods require vitamins and minerals from your diet to help process them. The more empty calorie foods you consume, the more you add to your nutritional deficiency.

Many older women do not want to cook anymore after their children have left home. Some men do not know how to cook. A high school boy working as a bagger at Stop & Shop told me that the healthy-looking senior citizens were those purchasing fruits and vegetables, meats and eggs and the sick looking ones hanging onto their shopping carts so they could stand up were junk foods and soda.

82. Some Bad Effects of Obesity

By: Dr. Judith Giustini

If you are obese, your heart has to work harder. Heart failure is more common amongst obese people. Obese people have more cancer than people of normal weight. For women, it's cancer of the breast, uterus and ovaries. For men, it's cancer of the colon, rectum and prostate. Obese people have more osteoarthritis, gout and gallbladder disease.

Obesity doubles or triples your risk of premature death. It is estimated that 300,000 deaths per year are caused by obesity. It could be more, if you count heart attacks. If obesity does not kill you, it can certainly make you miserable.

Many obese people have a poor body image, which leads to self-consciousness and discomfort in social situations. Obese people may experience prejudice and job discrimination, causing feelings of rejection and low self-esteem.

Dieting seems like a harsh punishment to an obese person who loves food. Each person has their food preferences and habits of indulging themselves. When you are obese, you can consume excess calories and maintain your elevated weight. When you lose weight, it will take fewer calories to maintain your weight.

Many people who succeed in losing weight on a 1,200 to 1,500 calorie diet, only to regain it again as soon as they stop the diet. Dieting must include permanent changes in your lifestyle choices. This project requires constant attention. The results can be worth it. Think about living the rest of your life as a normal-weight person!

83. Some of the Ways Sugar Ruins Your Health

From various Internet sources

By: Dr. Judith Giustini

In 1700, the average person consumed about four pounds of sugar per year. These days, many Americans are consuming more than one-half pound of sugar per day. Some negative things said by knowledgeable people are:

Excess consumption of sugar suppresses your immune system and this interferes with your ability to resist viruses and bacterial infections. It causes reactive hypoglycemia, which is pre-diabetic. Some symptoms of hypoglycemia are: hyperactivity, anxiety, difficulty concentrating and crankiness.

Excess consumption of sugar causes a rise in triglycerides. It also contributes to a loss of tissue elasticity and function, reduces high-density lipoproteins (causing "cholesterol" problems). It leads to deficiency of chromium and copper, and it interferes with the absorption of calcium and magnesium.

Excess consumption of sugar causes premature aging, leads to alcoholism, causes tooth decay and contributes to obesity. It is said to increase the risk of Crohn's disease, ulcerative colitis and gastric or duodenal ulcers, arthritis, and asthma and to assist in the uncontrolled growth of Candida yeast, cause gallstones, heart disease, appendicitis, multiple sclerosis, hemorrhoids, varicose veins, periodontal disease and osteoporosis. It upsets mineral relationships in the body. It can cause hyperactivity, anxiety, difficulty concentrating and crankiness in children.

In the past, it was thought that high cholesterol was caused by excess consumption of fats, but recent information has indicated that sugar is a cause, and that it also is involved in hardening of the arteries.

84. Stresses That Interfere with Dieting Success

By: Dr. Judith Giustini

Stress distracts your attention from paying attention to your diet and outs your body in the fight-flight mode.

<u>Chapter:</u>

85. More Stresses That Interfere with Dieting Success

By: Dr. Judith Giustini

In her book *Feelings Buried Alive Never Die,* Karol K. Truman provides a list of subconscious negative feelings that pertain to certain words that are used for obesity, such as:

<u>Obesity</u>: using food as a substitute for affection

<u>Fat</u>: Feel a need for protection, Hidden anger

<u>Overweight</u>: Unexpressed, inappropriate feelings

<u>Compulsive Overeating</u>: Obesity is symbol of power and a desire to throw one's weight around. (See complete listing: Ch. 168.)

These feelings may have been programmed into your subconscious mind when you were very young, Negative feelings cause your body to produce toxic chemicals and then to have to dispose of them. This is an additional job for your body, which is already dealing with stress.

Each of your negative and positive feelings have vibrations that emanate into the energy fields around your body, and they can travel vwet far, causing you to attract the negative health, happiness and success that are in harmony with them. If you believe you are a victim or a martyr, or if you have low self-esteem, your "bad luck" (obesity) will serve to validate your negative feelings about yourself.

If you suppress your negative feelings out of your conscious mind (10% of thinking) into your subconscious mind (90%of thinking), you are giving them power. They force you to be in defense physiology, (fight-or-flight), and you won't know why you feel so upset and fatigued, and your weight is out of control.

86. Stomach Surgery for Obesity

By: Dr. Judith Giustini

From Internet research:

If your Body Mass Index is 40 or above (very obese) and you have health conditions that are associated with obesity, such as sleep apnea, diabetes, osteoarthritis, GERD or high blood pressure, and you have not had success with diet and exercise, you might be a candidate for stomach surgery. 3 procedures:

<u>Vertical Banded Gastroplasty</u> in which staples are used to restrict the size of the part the stomach that can receive food to a pouch that will hold about one ounce. A band of special fabric bypasses the lower part of the stomach. The band causes a feeling of fullness and delays the emptying of food from the pouch. Cost: about $14,500.

<u>Gastric Bypass Surgery</u> in which the stomach is divided into a small upper pouch about the size of a walnut and a much larger "remnant pouch". The food you eat will no longer go into some parts of your stomach and small intestine. Can reduce the absorption of nutrients. Cost: about $23,000.

<u>Adjustable Gastric Band </u> in which a band is placed around the upper part of the stomach that forms a pouch that can hold about one ounce of food. Sterile saline water can be injected into the band or removed from it through a tube that is accessible through a device under the skin. This will tighten or loosen the band. You will continue to absorb the nutrients you consume. Cost: about $3,349.

Many people lose about half of their *excess* weight during the first year and continue to lose slowly during the second and third year. Fewer than 10% have complications.

87. Symptoms of Acidosis
By: Dr. Judith Giustini

"Acidosis" is a physiological condition that is caused by consuming "acid-ash" foods, such as meats, fish, poultry, eggs, dairy products, beans and grains.

Early in your life, you may seem energized, because the acid in your system makes you agitated. Maybe you channel this acid energy into productive work and you become known as a high achiever, but later on, you find your get up and go has got up and gone.

It is said that all diseases thrive in an acid body, so if you develop a chronic degenerative disease or cancer, it may be difficult for you to get well, because your body is trying to keep you alive in the acid milieu that you have provided, and it can't properly deal with the additional problem of your disease.

Dehydration contributes to acidosis, because your body can't dilute the acids, and they can cause you harm. Dehydration is said to be a major factor in depression and obesity. You may develop chronic fatigue, leg cramps or an "acid" personality.

It is not easy to change to a plant-based diet and to drink the right amount of water for yourself each day, but it is worth seriously working on it, so you can help yourself to aging "gracefully" and avoiding some of the so-called diseases that are actually the physiological manifestations of what your body is doing to try and keep you alive, while dealing with the adverse consequences of what you have been eating and drinking.

88. What You Think as a Cause of Interference with Your Health, Happiness and Success

By: Dr. Judith Giustini

What do you think and why do you think it? Maybe you can answer this question as it pertains to your conscious thoughts (10% of thinking), but your subconscious thoughts (90% of thinking) are going on 24/7 without your conscious awareness. There is a whole program that deals with the functioning of every cell in your body, and how they all work together for the purpose of your survival and the communication between The Power That Made Your Body and The Power That Runs Your Body.

Your belief system – that "stern parent" that is in charge of your "should" and "ought's". This information is based on what you experienced with your five senses (what you saw, what you heard, what you smelled, what you tasted and what you touched), plus what you learned by observing what was going on around you, plus your feelings about your experiences, plus the things your parents tried to teach you when you were very young.

In her book *Feelings Buried Alive Never Die,* Karol K. Truman says that certain subconscious negative feelings can cause certain illnesses. For example, in the section *"Probable Feelings Causing Ill-ness",* under ***"Heart Trouble:",*** she lists the subconscious negative feelings of: "Violating the laws of love knowingly or unknowingly, Feelings of compassion being blocked, Feelings of resentment and/or hurt, Not feeling approval from others, upsetting family problems, Has a difficult time forgiving (including self), Wanting a release from responsibility." In Mind-Body Therapy, you can learn about *your* subconscious feelings buried alive.

89. Symptoms of Dehydration From You're Not Sick, You're Thirsty! By Dr. F. Batmanghelidj, M.D.

By: Dr. Judith Giustini

Dr. Batmanghelidh says that many physiological conditions thought to be illnesses are actually signs of chronic dehydration.

Asthma & Allergies
High Blood Pressure
Coronary Heart Disease
Heart Attacks, Strokes
Obesity, Type 2 Diabetes
Poor Digestion, Poor Assimilation of food
Constipation, Colitis pain
Hiatal Hernia, Heartburn
Autoimmune Diseases,
Osteoarthritis, Back pain
Rheumatoid Arthritis
Attention Deficit Disorder
Brain Damage, Dementia, Alzheimer's disease
Headaches and migraines
Depression
Chronic Fatigue Syndrome
Dry and burning eyes
Glaucoma
Gout
Kidney Stones
Osteoporosis
Cancer Formation
Impotency, Low Libido

If you have one or some of these illnesses, are you dehydrated? To change What You Drink, you will need to discipline yourself.

90. Veggie Dining Made Simple

By: Dr. Judith Giustini

The average adult male burns about 2,500 calories per day and the average adult female burns about 2,000 calories per day. If you consume 500 calories fewer than you burn, you will lose one lb. in 7 days. If you consume 1,500 calories per day (male)or 1,200 calories per day (female), you will lose about 2 lbs. per week.

You might have to keep doing this diet for quite a while, so it should be high in nutrients, low in calories and easy for you to follow. Choose a plant-based diet that is ideally 80% fruits and vegetables and 20% everything else.

A well-known weight loss group says you don't have to count the calories in most vegetables, and you can eat extra apples, boneless skinless chicken breast and hard-boiled eggs and still lose weight, but consider the source. This is the same group that is now recommending diet pills.

Maybe you are not a big fan of fruits and vegetables, but if they are in the Super Shakes (Ch.165.) that you prepare quickly and easily on your bender or in your Super Soups (Ch. 164.) which are delicious, but messy and time-consuming to make, but nice to have in your freezer. You need a diet that you enjoy, and that you will not mind coming back to whenever the need arises. Learn about the nutritional content of your foods.

Many people on this. diet use 4-5 eggs per day – 2-3 in their Shakes and 2 for a meal. Eggs are very nutritious, and they provide satiety (a feeling of fullness), which keeps you from just grabbing anything to eat that's handy. Beans are also good for this. Count the calories.

91. The 1,200 to 1,500 Calorie Diet

By: Dr. Judith Giustini

The more pounds you weigh, the more calories it takes you to maintain your weight. A man who weighs 300 lbs. will need to consume about 5,000 calories per day to maintain that weight, whereas a man who weighs 150 lbs. will only need to consume 2,500 to maintain that weight. If you consume 3,500 fewer calories per week than it takes to maintain your weight, you will lose 1 lb. So, if you consume 1,000 calories per day fewer than you burn for one week, you will lose 2 lbs. If you are obese, you will lose weight faster at the beginning.

One popular weight loss diet allows 2 slices of bread, 2 Tbs. fats 6 oz. protein and 3 fruits per day. You need to count the calories in pasta, rice, potatoes and beans, but most vegetables are unlimited, and you are allowed to have extra apples, boneless skinless chicken breast and hard-boiled eggs and still be on your diet. Before you start cutting calories, write down everything you consume for three days and add up the calories. Many people have reached their goal weight on this diet, but they don't want to return to it, because it is cumbersome, and they did not feel satisfied, so they don't want to return to it if they gain weight.

Your body was designed to run on a plant-based diet. People only began consuming animal flesh after the flood of Noah's day. Every cell in your body needs certain nutrients to function optimally. The alkaline diet is excellent for the health of your cells.

Dehydration is known to be a cause of obesity. In his book *Obesity Cancer Depression,* he recommends Dr. F. Batmanghelidj says you need to drink ½ ounce of water every day for every pound you weigh, and use 1 tsp. of sea salt for every gallon of water. If you are chronically dehydrated, your kidneys may be compromised. Maybe you can stick to 64 oz. per day?

92. The Dilemma of Obesity

By: Dr. Judith Giustini

If you are 100-200 lbs. overweight, you are considered to be severely obese. If you are more than 200 lbs. overweight, you are considered to be morbidly obese.

Obesity can shorten the number of days you are alive on the planet because heart disease, strokes, diabetes and cancer are common in obese people. Obesity can make you miserable every second of the day and night while you are here. Despite the prevalence of overweight people in our society, fat people often experience social and workplace discrimination.

There are so many obstacles to losing weight – customs, habits, associations, prevalence of high-calorie foods, lack of availability of nutritious food, lack of knowledge about appropriate diet, inability to exercise, inertia, discouragement, diabetes, hypoglycemia, etc.

Obesity is a terrible affliction. What is causing it may be more than consuming too many calories. We need to find out what is motivating you to overeat. If you have a history of adverse childhood (or adult) experiences, you may have many unresolved negative feelings buried alive in your subconscious mind, tormenting you, making you turn to food for solace.

The dilemma of obesity is that there are so many aspects to it, and that it can seem impossible to deal with enough of them at the same time for you to succeed in your quest for a normal size body, so maybe you just give up trying. You may need help to get you from Confusion to Clarity to Focus to Peace, so you can take charge of things in your life.

93. She Had the Yo-Yo Weight Syndrome

By: Dr. Judith Giustini

A woman, who was a famous TV personality, got tired of being obese, and she went on a liquid protein diet and lost a significant amount of weight. She was delighted to be able to fit into size 8 jeans, and she posed in them on TV But a liquid protein diet is not a prescription that leads to living in a normal weight body for the long term, and she gradually regained all the weight she had lost, plus a few more pounds.

She hired a nutritionist, a cook and a personal trainer, but she also had a penchant for fast foods and batter fried chicken. It was a constant battle that sometimes she was winning and sometimes she was losing. In her business, she had to eat out frequently with associates, and her weight went up and downlike a yo-yo.

From time to time, she would go on another fad diet, and get her weight back down to somewhat normal, but then the holidays would come along . . . She decided to get serious about dieting, so he joined a famous weight loss group. Some people lose 2 lbs. per week on this diet, but it took her 2 years to reach a somewhat normal bodyweight.

When the weight loss group started offering diet pills, she started using them, and she lost a great deal of weight. Hopefully, she won't have the same experience as many dieters, of regaining the weight gradually, after stopping using the pills.

Many folks who struggle with their weight due to the stress of subconscious negative feelings have found help in Mind-Body Therapy (Ch. 126.)

94. Underlying Causes of Excess Bodyweight

By: Dr. Judith Giustini

People who have never had to watch their weight often judge their pudgy fellow humans as being uncaring or irresponsible about themselves. They probably don't know how much work some people have gone to trying to lose weight, only to end up fat again.

There are many reasons why it is so difficult to lose those extra pounds. These include eating too much and exercising too little. This gets worse if you have a sedentary lifestyle and/or a disability that prevents you from exercising. Then there are the effects of your habits. You eat what you eat because that's the way you have always done it, or that is the custom you grew up with. If you get hungry, angry, lonely, or tired, this can drive you to overeating or overdrinking. Once you are free of the subconscious mind chatter that has been distracting you from paying attention to this joy-killing, life-threatening problem of obesity, you will be taking steps towards health, happiness and success.

Once you understand the cause of your negative feelings and forgive those persons who are involved in it(including yourself), you will have removed some Obstacles to Healing (being well/normal size) you will have moved a few more steps towards taking charge of things in your life.

95. How You Rest as a Cause of Interference with Your Health, Happiness and Success

By: Dr. Judith Giustini

How you rest affects the physiology of every cell in your body, especially your nervous system. When you are sleeping, your body should be in the Parasympathetic ("breed and feed") mode. If you don't sleep well, your body is not going to have the right kind of "down time", so it can do its job of cleansing and healing your cells and tissues.

If you have Insomnia, why is that? In her book *Feelings Buried Alive Never Die,* Karol K. Truman lists under "Probable Feelings Causing Illness.

Insomnia: Tensions in life, Deep seeded guilt, Feelings of fear & anxiety, Reaction to potential threatening situations, worrying about being able/good enough to do what is needed to be done" Sleep deprivation interferes with your ability to think complicated thoughts and contributes to weight gain. You go through your day not feeling truly alert. Maybe you get grouchy. Maybe your body grabs a few winks at an inconvenient time (driving, sitting in a meeting . . .).

If how you rest is "not-so-good", this can certainly be a cause of interference with your health, happiness, and success.

What to do: If the feelings that are causing your insomnia are buried in your subconscious mind, you may not know what they are, and you may be in Confusion. Maybe you would benefit from a Mind-Body Therapy Search. However, you do have access to your conscious mind. Is there somebody you have not apologized to? somebody who still owes you an apology? Can you apologize to them or forgive yourself and everybody else connected with the situation? Can you forgive them anyway?

96. Water Deficiency and Other Links to Ill-ness

By: Dr. Judith Giustini

If you or somebody you know have/has allergies, asthma, Alzheimer's disease, constipation, diabetes, fatigue, heart attack, hypertension, obesity or quite a few other "diseases", you might be surprised to learn that there is a common cause associated with all of them, which is chronic dehydration. See: *You're Not Sick, You're Thirsty* by Dr. F. Batmanghelidj who says, "Don't treat thirst with medications". (watercure.com)

You might think that once you know how much water you should be drinking every day it would be easy just to do it, but this is not so. You need to *discipline* yourself to drink your water. The power of your habits can be difficult to overcome.

Dr. M. T. Morter, Jr., M.S., D.C. taught that type 2 diabetes and many other conditions were linked to acid/alkaline balance related to diet. He recommended a diet that was 80% fruits and vegetables and 20% proteins and other foods, which is similar to the diet that Dr. F. Batmanghelidj recommends in his book *Obesity Cancer Depression.*

97. What the Experts Say about Diet for Proper Weight

By: Dr. Judith Giustini

Dr. F. Batmanghelidj, in *Your Body's Many Cries for Water,* says that your brain needs the energy from the hydroelectricity of water and from sugar in your blood circulation. It is easy to mistake the feeling of thirst for the feeling of hunger and eat food when you should be drinking water, thus causing yourself to gain weight. He says that "fluids" are not the same thing as water.

Dr. M. T. Morter, Jr., in *An Apple a Day,* says that excess dietary protein causes acid pH, which results in diabetes. He recommends a diet of 80% fruits and vegetables, which is also a diet that helps you to maintain a proper bodyweight.

Dr. Joel Fuhrman in *Eat to live, The End of Diabetes,* says your diet should be high in nutrients and low in calories.

Dr. Daniel Amen, in *Change Your Brain, Change Your Body,* says that to lose weight and stay healthy for life, you need to focus on fruits and vegetables.

Dr. Mark Hyman says to avoid refined foods. He says there's no such thing as junk food. There's junk and there's food.

On the Weight Watchers diet, you have 3 fruits per day and most vegetables are unlimited.

Trimdownclub.com says never to consume concentrated orange juice, wheat, high fructose corn syrup, and tofu.

98. Your Amazing Adrenal Glands

By: Dr. Judith Giustini

Your adrenal glands are small endocrine glands that sit atop your kidneys. They secrete hormones that regulate your blood pressure, your metabolism and your electrolyte balance. The androgen they secrete is converted to functional sex hormones in your gonads. In a situation of perceived harmful threat, attack, or threat to survival, they produce epinephrine and norepinephrine, which work with your nervous system in your fight-or-flight response.

Other causes of stress are deficiencies of nutrients. Nutrients are the basis of the health of every cell and tissue in your body and all of the hormones, enzymes, neurotransmitters, etc. People who use heroin lose the sensations of hunger and thirst. People who seek out such substances may be doing so as a response to stress. Then they have the additional stress of getting a regular supply of the drug after they get addicted.

Chronic dehydration is a threat to your survival that causes chronic stress. Your adrenal glands do not plan or think. They respond to stimuli. Chronic stress can overwhelm your adrenal glands. You will feel exhausted, low in libido, your blood pressure may become elevated and you may be vulnerable to bacteria and viruses.

You can have chronic stress from negative feelings stored in your subconscious mind (90% of thinking). The events that generated these feelings might be deep in your memories. You *believe* that you have dealt with them, but if you have not resolved your negative feelings, they are still very much alive and they need to be identified, replaced and forgiven.

99. How to be Your Adrenal Glands' Best Friend

By: Dr. Judith Giustini

Your adrenal glands are central to the digestive and hormonal functions of your body. They balance the function of your nerve fibers. They work in concert with your pituitary gland to oxidize the free fatty acids in your adipose tissue.

<u>Your adrenal glands need</u>:

<u>HYDRATION</u>: If you don't drink enough water, your fight-or-flight reaction to this emergency makes your body focused on survival, rather than health. A time-honored recommendation for adults is 64 oz. of water per day for adults. If you have been dehydrated for a long time, you need to increase your intake of water gradually, so as not to overwhelm your kidneys.

<u>NUTRIENTS</u>: Your adrenal glands are greatly influenced by a hormone from your pituitary gland that activates them. Vitamin A, Vitamin C, vitamin D, Niacin, Pantothenic Acid and Biotin, plus sixteen amino acids and a full array of trace minerals are needed to build this hormone.

<u>pH</u>: Every function to your body is sensitive to the pH you create in it through your choices of what you eat, drink and think. If your pH is "off", your adrenal glands will be stressed.

<u>STRESS RELIEF</u>: In her book *Feelings Buried Alive Never Die*, Karol K Truman lists feelings that cause adrenal problems, some of which are: "Feeling defeated, feeling like a victim, lack of courage, feelings of anxiety, unresolved jealousies and fears."

100

100. Your Amazing Brain

By: Dr. Judith Giustini

Your nervous system is made up of your brain, your spinal cord and your peripheral nerves. Your nerve cells communicate with one another electrically and biochemically.

Your brain is the resource of all your thoughts, feelings, beliefs and moods. Your brain is the control center for the rest of your body. Your brain coordinates your ability to see, hear, touch, taste, and smell. Your brain enables you to understand and communicate in words, to do mathematics, to appreciate music, to plan ahead, and to fantasize.

Your brain reviews the stimuli from your internal organs, the surface of your body and your eyes, ears, nose and mouth. It uses this information to govern the position of your limbs, the rate of functioning of your internal organs and the state of your mood, consciousness and alertness.

Your beautiful, complex nervous system is unfortunately vulnerable to many diseases and injuries. It is subject to infections of bacteria or viruses. It is subject to strokes due to blockages in the blood supply and to degenerative diseases such as Alzheimer's disease or Parkinson's disease.

Your brain can become traumatized by injury, such as in warfare, accidents, or sports. Tumors can cause structural damage to your brain and spinal cord. Your brain needs constant oxygen and nourishment. At all times, about 20% of the blood flow from your heart is flowing through your brain.

101. How to Be Your Brain's Best Friend

By: Dr. Judith Giustini

Your brain receives nutrients through your bloodstream. Your blood-brain barrier blocks many toxic substances from entering your brain, except for alcohol, caffeine, antidepressants and cannabinoids. Methamphetamine, cocaine and nicotine are said to alter the function of the blood-brain barrier and allow the invasion of bacteria and viruses into the brain.

HYDRATION: In his book *Your Body's Many Cries for Water*, Dr. F. Batmanghelidj says that dehydrated people often suffer from fear, anxiety and depression and they may become antisocial, suicidal or homicidal. This is because dehydration interferes with the electrical energy-generating effects of water. Drink your water and be your brain's friend.

NUTIENTS: Dr. Batmanghelidj recommends one-half teaspoon of unrefined sea salt for every two quarts of water you drink. He says that low intake of salt can be an initiating factor for cancer. He says that our diet should contain plenty of fruits and vegetables because they supply natural water-soluble vitamins and minerals that are usable by the cells of your brain and body.

Scientists say that your body was designed to run most efficiently at a slightly alkaline state, where your urine has a pH of about 7.0, based on a diet high in fruits and vegetables. Animal proteins and grains create an acid pH, which, along with dehydration, can lead to neurological disorders such as Alzheimer's disease or Parkinson's disease. You can learn to check your urine pH to see how you are doing with your diet.

102. Your Amazing Heart

By: Dr. Judith Giustini

Your heart is an organ about the size of your fist, and it usually weighs about 10 0unces.It sits behind your breastbone, between your lungs. Your heart receives oxygen-poor blood from your body, pumps it to the lungs to be oxygenated, receives it back, and pumps it out through your arteries to your cells, and back to your heart through your veins. Your heart beats over 100,000 times per day, and pumps about 5,000 gallons of blood throughout your body.

Your nervous system sends signals that tell your heart to beat faster during activity and slower during rest. Your endocrine system sends out hormones that tell your blood vessel walls to relax or constrict, and this affects your blood pressure.

Your heart's valves are like doors between your upper and lower heart chambers. The tricuspid valve is the door between your right atrium and right ventricle, and the mitral valve is the door between your left atrium and left ventricle. Your Pulmonary valve opens to receive oxygen-poor blood from your right ventricle into your pulmonary arteries. Your Aortic valve opens when oxygenated blood flows out of your left ventricle into your aorta to go to your body.

Your heart receives nutrients through the coronary arteries that run along your heart's surface. It has an electrical conduction system that is like the wiring system of a house.

103. How to be Your Heart's Best Friend

By: Dr. Judith Giustini

Some common conditions seen by cardiovascular specialists are:

Atrial fibrillation: due to irregular electrical impulses
Arrhythmia: heartbeat too fast, too slow or irregular
Congestive heart failure: heart muscle too stiff or weak
Coronary artery disease: plaque narrows arteries
Heart attack: sudden blockage of coronary arteries

Your heart is working for your survival 24/7. You can help by

What you eat (Ch. 53.): Your heart needs vital nutrients that mostly come from plant-based sources.

What you drink) Ch. 43.): Dehydration is a major cause of heart trouble and high blood pressure. See: *Your Body's Many Cries for Water* by Dr. F. Batmanghelidj. Drink alcohol in moderation. Limit intake of caffeine.

What you breathe (Ch. 89.) Your lungs are composed of delicate tissues that can be injured by har0sh chemicals such as nicotine.

How you exercise (Ch. 43).: You need to spend about 150 minutes per week doing moderate exercise.

How you rest (Ch. 170.): When you are sleeping is when your body does it's housekeeping jobs. One of the best things you can do for your heart is to keep your weight where it is supposed to be.

What you think (Ch. 171.): Feelings such as: Feelings of rejection, resentment or hurt, feeling unloved, disapproved of, upsetting relationships, want to get away, or upsetting financial, work, living situations can distract you from taking charge of things in your life (like your weight loss program).

104. Your Amazing Kidneys

By: Dr. Judith Giustini

Your two kidneys are situated on the back part of your abdomen, one on each side of your vertebral column. They are about four inches high and two inches wide. Each kidney contains about 2,000,000 tubules, the total length of which is about 75 miles. Your kidneys continuously produce urine, which drains into your bladder through your ureters. From your bladder, the urine drains through your urethra and exits your body.

The primary functions of your kidneys are to filter your blood and excrete waste products. They selectively reabsorb water, glucose and amino acids and help to regulate your blood pressure by maintaining salt and water balance. Your kidneys produce a hormone that stimulates the growth of red blood cells in your bone marrow, helping to maintain the health of your bones through converting Vitamin D to calcitriol, which stimulates absorption of calcium and phosphorous from your small intestine and helping to regulate your acid/alkaline balance.

After the age of 30 to 40, most people's kidneys become less efficient at filtering blood. Many older people experience urinary incontinence and they end up in nursing homes because of falls while rushing to use the toilet.

Some symptoms of kidney dysfunction are: fatigue, nausea, vomiting, swelling of ankles and feet, low back pain and body odor. Your kidneys are affected by toxins, such as drugs, alcohol, tobacco smoke, vitamin overdoses, shellfish and pork. Dehydration is very hard on your kidneys.

105. How to Be Your Kidneys' Best Friend

By: Dr. Judith Giustini

You want your kidneys to work quietly and uneventfully. Dialysis twice a week can't be any fun.

Your kidneys need:

HYDRATION: At any given time, 20% of your blood is going through your kidneys. A long-time recommendation from medical doctors has been 64 oz. per day, however some authorities recommend ½ oz. of water per lb. bodyweight.

NUTRIENTS: Your body was designed to utilize nutrients from natural sources – vitamin A from carrots or fish liver oils, etc. Supplements of natural trace elements may be helpful.

pH: If you eat a lot of high protein foods, this produces an acid condition in your body, which strains your kidneys in their effort to maintain your acid/alkaline balance, especially if you are dehydrated.

Certain negative feelings, such as concern about survival issues, repressed emotions and criticism of others have been noted as prevalent amongst people who have kidney problems. So you could drink the right amount of water and stick to the best diet of organic whole foods and still be having problems with your kidneys due to the unresolved negative feelings running constantly in your subconscious mind causing trouble with your kidneys. You can forgive them if you know what they are.

106. Your Amazing Large Intestine

By: Dr. Judith Giustini

Your large intestine (large bowel or colon) is the last stop in your digestive system before your waste exits your body through your anus. Your large intestine starts in the lower right side of your abdomen at the cecum where your small intestine ends. Your appendix is located on the lower part of your cecum. Your large intestine is about 4.9 feet long. After your cecum is your ascending colon, your transverse colon and your descending colon, your rectum and your anus.

The function of your large intestine is to absorb water from the remaining indigestible food matter and then to pass useless waste material out of your body. The waste you eliminate is not solely from food. Every cell of your body is like a little person. It ingests and it excretes. Tissue wastes, dead blood cells and dead bacteria are included in your feces.

Your large intestine contains about 700 species of friendly bacteria that perform a variety of functions such as breaking down fibers and producing large amounts of vitamins, especially Vitamin K, which is important in blood clotting, and the B vitamin Biotin. Taking antibiotics that kill good bacteria can lead to vitamin deficiency and irritation that causes excess secretion of mucus and leads to diarrhea.

It takes your large intestine about 16 hours to finish up processing the food you ate. Intestinal contents are liquid when they enter your large intestine, but semi-solid when they reach your rectum as stool.

Constipation can result from dehydration or medications.

107. How to be Your Large Intestine's Best Friend

By: Dr. Judith Giustini

When your large intestine is not working properly, you can experience symptoms: constipation, diarrhea alternating with constipation, foul smelling stools, fatigue, hemorrhoids, diverticulitis and varicose veins.

At least 30% of the people you know have infrequent bowel movements that are difficult to pass (constipation). The most common cause of constipation is dehydration. If you are constipated, try drinking 2 glasses of water when you get up and 2 glasses of water before breakfast. Having your impacted feces manually removed in the hospital is probably not fun.

<u>Your Large Intestine needs</u>:

<u>HYDRATION</u>: Most of the functions of your digestive system take place in water, especially in your large intestine. Dehydration is an emergency that will block losing weight.

<u>NUTRITION</u>: Your colon is a muscle. If you are malnourished and dehydrated, your starving muscles can't work well. If you are trying to lose weight, you might have to work on getting your cells healthy before you can lose weight.

<u>pH</u>: Foods which leave an acid ash after they are burned in your body are: animal flesh, eggs, dairy, etc. Acid eating leads to "acid personality" (crankiness). Fruits and vegetables leave an alkaline ash that is favorable to long-term wellness.

<u>STRESS RELIEF</u>: Subconscious feelings such as parsimony, lying to self or others or anxiety can upset your large intestine.

108. Your Amazing Liver

By: Dr. Judith Giustini

Your liver is a large organ that lies underneath your ribs on the right side of your body. After the nutrients of the food, you ate are absorbed into the capillaries of your small intestine and portal circulation, they are delivered to your liver for processing. In your liver, where bacteria and foreign particles are removed, and the nutrients are processed. After several hours, blood, now laden with nutrients, leaves your liver and goes into your general circulation to feed your cells.

Your liver has many functions:

BLOOD: Your liver regulates your blood volume. It supplies all the elements for blood formation. Vitamins A, B, D and K are synthesized in your liver. Your liver also produces substances for blood clotting.

DETOXIFICATION: Your liver destroys noxious materials, viruses, bacteria and metabolic waste. It works with your immune system.

METABOLISM: Your liver produces glucose from your diet and stores it as glycogen. When glucose is needed in your body, your liver changes the glycogen to glucose and releases it into your blood stream.

Hormones from your pancreas influence your liver to store glycogen. Hormones from your adrenals influence your liver to release glucose. Your liver synthesizes amino acids (proteins) and uric acid. Your liver absorbs minerals, which serve to balance your pH. Your liver secretes bile.

109. How to be Your Liver's Best Friend

By: Dr. Judith Giustini

<u>Your Liver needs:</u>

OXYGEN: Your liver needs fresh, oxygenated blood. Lack of oxygen due to air pollution (smoking) impairs liver function.

HYDRATION: Your bloodstream is called "The River of Life". Your blood carries nutrients to all the cells of your body. In dehydration, your body borrows water from your blood. Dehydration impairs your liver function (and more).

pH: A diet that is 75-80% fruits and vegetables and 20-25%nuts, whole grains and minimal animal proteins helps your body maintain a healthy pH. The activity of enzymes, coenzymes, vitamins and minerals are affected by pH Alkaline pH facilitates the chemistry you need.

AVOIDING LIVER TOXINS: According to Edward F. Schwartz, Ph.D., in his book *Endocrines, Organs and their Impact,* substances to be avoided are: Coffee, coffee-mate, black tea, alcohol, soft drinks, white flour, canned goods, candy, deep fried foods, chocolate, mayonnaise, heated fats, boxed cereals, food colorings, rich gravies, milk, meat and fish (use infrequently) unripe fruits, hard boiled eggs.

RESOLVE NEGATIVE FEELINGS

In her book *Feelings Buried Alive Never Die,* Karol K. Truman says that The liver is the Anger Center and that feelings such as: Unresolved anger, resentment, pettiness, Being judgmental, Critical thoughts, Not forgiving self & others, Feelings of injustice & revenge, Regret over the past and Sadness can cause liver problems.

110. Your Amazing Pancreas

By: Dr. Judith Giustini

Your pancreas is an organ about six inches long, shaped like a dog's tongue. It lies beneath your lower ribs on the left side of your abdomen. Your pancreas secretes enzymes and a bicarbonate solution into your small intestine for digestion. It also secretes insulin. Insulin promotes the utilization of glucose in muscle and fat tissues. Your pancreas works in concert with your pituitary gland, your adrenals, your liver and your nervous system.

The enzymes your pancreas produces are built from amino acids (proteins). Enzymes are important in digesting your foods and as anti-inflammatory agents. Inflammation is caused by stress due to cuts, bruises, food reactions, chemical reactions, heat, cold, anger and anxiety. Pancreatic enzymes have been called Nature's Tranquilizers.

If your pancreas is not working properly, you might experience pain on the inside of your left shoulder blade, pain on the left side of your abdomen, headache relieved by eating, waking up and can't get back to sleep, emotional storms on empty stomach, indigestion 2 hours after eating, asthma, allergies, arthritic pain with swelling, shingles on trunk of body, white spots on fingernails, constipation, dryness of skin, diabetes, boils and chronic infections, psychoses, learning disabilities and autism. Pancreatic enzyme supplements are available. Your pancreas is an important player on your weight loss team because of its role in digestion and maintaining stable blood sugar.

111. How to be Your Pancreas' Best Friend

By: Dr. Judith Giustini

It is important to treat your pancreas kindly, because there are consequences if you don't. Some pancreatic problems are:

A gallstone blocking the common duct to your intestine, causing pancreatic enzymes to back up and begin to digest the cells of your pancreas, resulting in severe inflammation. Gallstones are related to consuming excess acid foods (meats, dairy, fish, grains) and stress. Chronic alcoholism can cause the small ducts in your pancreas to clog, resulting in acute pancreatitis. Overeating is a strain on your pancreas.

<u>You can help your pancreas serve you well by</u>: According to Dr. F. Batmanghelidj, in his book *Your Body's Many Cries for Water,* non-insulin diabetes is most probably the result of a water-deficiency that causes your brain to peg-up your glucose threshold so it can meet its needs for sugar. Water and salt are essential for the generation of hydroelectric energy and for neurotransmitter mechanisms.

<u>NUTRITION</u>: Tryptophan, an amino acid from egg whites, raw soybeans, pumpkin seeds, and fish, is important in diabetes and cancer prevention. The alkaline nutrients of fruits and vegetables support your pancreas' health.

<u>FORGIVE NEGATIVE FEELINGS</u>: Pancreas problems are often related to unresolved subconscious negative feelings of judgment, guilt, and low self-esteem. Diabetes is believed to be related to feelings of joylessness, and shame.

112

112. Your Amazing Small Intestine

By: Dr. Judith Giustini

Your small intestine is composed of three sections: the duodenum, the jejunum and the ileum. After digestion in your stomach, the food is released into your duodenum in amounts that your small intestine can process. This food receives enzymes from your pancreas that that work on proteins and bile from your gall bladder that works on the fats.

Digested foods enter the jejunum and the ileum and are absorbed into your blood steam through your intestinal walls and the nutrients travel to your liver for further processing and release into your blood stream to be transported to your cells. The waste products empty into your large intestine.

In gastric bypass surgery, rows of staples are used to divide the stomach into two parts. One part is a small pouch where the food from the diet goes for digestion. The lower part of the stomach and the upper part of the small intestine are bypassed and the upper part of the stomach is attached to the small intestine, so that digestive juices from the duodenum can reach the rest of the small intestine and be mixed with food.

Many people have lost weight following gastric bypass surgery, only to regain it gradually afterwards because they indulge in sugary snacks, sodas and alcohol. These items do not spend long in the stomach, so the person does not feel full. The person also may not feel nourished. Because they are not getting the nutrients out of their food, they may become hypoglycemic or diabetic, or they may become very hungry due to malnutrition, and they may keep eating small amounts of food frequently and gain weight. If the foods they choose are low in nutrients, they may aggravate their malnutrition.

113. How to be Your Small Intestine's Best Friend

By: Dr. Judith Giustini

Your small intestine is the next step in digestion after partially digested food leaves your stomach. In the first part of your small intestine, your food is mixed with copious amounts of a bicarbonate-containing solution from your pancreas that neutralizes the acid from your stomach and enzymes from your pancreas. Your gallbladder also secretes bile into your small intestine to emulsify fats.

HYDRATION: The process of digestion is a big user of water. Everything you consume into your digestive system can become a poison if it is not properly digested. Dehydration forces your body to borrow water from other important functions. It is important for you to drink two glasses of water one half-hour before each meal, because almost all of this water goes into your digestive juices.

NUTRITION: Your small intestine is composed of many specialized cells, such as the muscle cells that provide peristalsis to churn the intestinal contents and move them along. Your small intestine also contains cells that secrete mucus and villi and microvilli that absorb digested food into your bloodstream. For good digestion, it is important that these tissues are in good health. They need nutrients from the foods you eat, digest, absorb and utilize.

STRESS: In her book *Feelings Buried Alive Never Die,* Karol K. Truman says that **Indigestion** is often associated with: Feelings that everyone is against you, feeling you need to fight your way through life, Feelings of anxiety, Fear of losing job, losing security and/or Lack of understanding what, how, when, where or why in life.

114. What is Causing Your Stress?

By: Dr. Judith Giustini

Maybe your stress is coming from an illness, a disability, people in your home-life or work-life, your living situation, credit card debt, school loans, fear of the future, emotional baggage, PTSD, etc. Stress causes your body to be running in the fight-or-flight mode, and you can end up in Exhaustion. The next step is the nursing home.

Maybe you are bringing stress upon yourself by what you choose to eat and drink. If you eat foods that are high in calories and low in nutrients, you are giving your body the problem of making do with whatever paltry amount and quality of vitamins and minerals you have provided. If your diet also is high in calories, your body will store the excess in your fat cells. You will be doing "Starvation in the Midst of Plenty".

In his book *You're Not Sick, You're Thirsty,* Dr. F. Batmanghelidj shows that many so-called "illnesses" are caused by what the person's body is doing physiologically in response to dehydration.

Another kind of stress you might not think about much is the stress of the negative feelings that you have suppressed (maybe embarrassing, maybe "just too awful". These feelings are not gone. They are buried alive in your subconscious mind, where they still have power over you. Also, they are sending out vibrations into your energy fields and these vibrations act according to The Law of Attraction, bringing you those very things you say you ***don't*** want - maybe confirming some negative beliefs about our self – and surely interfering with your health, happiness, and success.

115. What is Your Goal Weight?

By: Dr. Judith Giustini

Appropriate bodyweight for a woman 5 feet tall is said to be 100 lbs., and 5 lbs. more for every inch taller, so the bodyweight for a woman 5'7" tall should be 135 lbs. There is a similar appropriate bodyweight for men. There is a mathematical formula of how many calories per day you need to "un-eat" or exercise off in order for you to lose 1lb. The problem is: doing it.

There are many obstacles between where you might be right now and reaching your goal weight. If you were obese as a child, you may have 5 times more fat cells than a person who was a normal weight child. Then the is the influence of what people eat in your culture, plus the goodies you have become accustomed to (and feel deprived if you don't get them), plus the effect of lack of exercise.

Obesity is a terrible problem. These days, with so much company of others whose weight is out of control, it might not feel like such a stigma, but it can definitely interfere with your health, happiness and success. The bad thing is that you are the one who is causing it. The good thing is that you are the one who has the power to make it go away.

If you choose to reach your goal weight, there are many obstacles you will have to overcome. One obstacle could be lack of knowledge. How many calories are you allowed to eat each day for your weight loss diet and for your maintenance diet once you reach your goal weight?

116. Why is it So Difficult to Change Your Habits?

By: Dr. Judith Giustini

What you eat and drink may *seem* to be conscious choices, but actually, they are controlled by a subconscious system that is working to help you survive from microsecond to microsecond.

This system has to prioritize its efforts – some here, some there – whatever is the most important thing to focus on when it is trying to keep you alive – respiration, cardiac, digestion, elimination, etc. You may not be providing the ideal selection of nutrients and you might not be drinking enough water. You are living under stress, and you still have a bundle of stress from before.

Maybe you are unaware that an ideal diet is 80% fruits and vegetables. Maybe you didn't know that pork and scavengers are forbidden in The Bible because they are deleterious to your health. Maybe you didn't know that you need to drink at least 64 oz. of water per day. Maybe you have picked up some unhealthy habits – tobacco, drugs, alcohol . . .

You might think you could easily change your food and drink choices, but *nope*. Your habits are rooted in the subconscious belief system that was established in you when you were very young. It is like a stern parent that tells you how things are "supposed" to be. It might be programmed wrong.

If you keep doing the same things over again, according to your eating, drinking, and thinking habits, and your symptoms keep getting worse, maybe it's time to re-evaluate what you are doing. Habits are stubborn. Change may require a struggle.

117. "You Are Not Sick, You Are Thirsty"

By: Dr. Judith Giustini

"YOU ARE NOT SICK, YOU ARE THIRSTY! Don't treat thirst with medications" That is what it says on the cover of Dr. F. Batmanghelidj's book *Your Body's Many Cries For Water.* He also wrote the book *You Are Not Sick, You Are Thirsty!* and his tapes and other writings are offered on his websitewatercure.com

Dr. Batmanghelidj says that chronic cellular dehydration is a cause of premature death, and that the physiological manifestations of dehydration have been labeled as "diseases of unknown origin". He says that medications are palliatives, not designed to cure degenerative diseases.

In *Your Body's Many Cries for Water,* he discusses the relationship between dehydration and digestive problems, arthritis, back and neck pain, heart trouble, high blood pressure, diabetes, high cholesterol and obesity.

It is important for you to learn how much water you should be drinking each and every day, and for you to learn to overcome the habits that caused your dehydration.

A rather pudgy woman, visibly uncomfortable sitting in a chair, waiting for her turn in the blood lab, said that years ago, she had made a practice of drinking 2 quarts of water per day, and her weight was 35 lbs. less than now, and her back did not hurt. Since she has been under the control of her old habits, she got fat again and her back hurts.

118. You Can Choose to Avoid Empty Calories

By: Dr. Judith Giustini

Empty calories . . . sweet, crunchy, delicious . . . as your weight creeps up.

Every cell and tissue of your body requires nutrients from plant-based sources to keep your bones strong, your digestion happening, your brain working, etc. Your body will do the best it can, considering the nutritional circumstances you provide for it. but it will eventually break down due to deprivation.

Empty calories, such as sugar, white flour, excess fats and alcohol require vitamins and minerals from your diet to process them. If you are an empty calorie diet, you are causing your nutritional deficiencies. When your organ systems break down, your body will lack the nutritional building blocks to repair our cells.

If you are also consuming more calories than it takes to maintain your weight, you will gain one pound/3,500 excess calories. So easy to gain, so hard to lose! ("A moment on the lips, a lifetime on the hips")

You can choose to avoid empty calories, but what are you going to replace them with? The experts are saying you need to consume 80% fruits and vegetables. Dehydration is a major cause of obesity. Many people have reported a significant weight loss after starting to drink the right amount water each day.

How about if you start out by just avoiding white sugar and white flour and drinking 64 ounces of water per day?

119. Your Calories and Your Weight

By: Dr. Judith Giustini

People from places where food is scarce are usually skinny. Fashion models keep their weight low by eating hardly anything. Looking around, it seems as if there is not a famine in the USA today.

Body weight is tricky. It sneaks up on you when you are not looking. A few snacks here, some little treats there . . . a couple of extra pounds a year. If you overeat by 3,500 calories, you gain a pound. That could be 10 calories one day and 100 calories the next day. It all adds up.

Each person burns a certain number of calories per day, depending on their weight and their lifestyle. The more you weigh, the more calories it takes for you to walk around and breathe air. When you lose weight, it will take fewer calories to maintain you at your new lower weight. When you look in the mirror and you are surprised about how big you have become, you might decide to "do something". Doing something radical – like skipping meals or going on a fast are non-solutions to your problem. They might work for a few days, but then, no. When you start back eating, you may eat more because you feel deprived and you need a reward.

For long-term living in a normal-weight body, you need to learn to control your calories. Not all calories are created equal. Fruits and vegetables, beans, and brown rice contain vital nutrients. To lose weight, you need to feed yourself, not starve yourself. Dr. F. Batmanghelidj in *Your Body's Many Cries for Water* recommends 2 glasses of water ½ hour before each meal to help your body make your digestive juices

120. Your Fat Contains Whaaat?

By: Dr. Judith Giustini

An article called "Fat" in Wikipedia says that your body uses your fat as a place to store disease organisms and toxic chemicals from your diet until they can be removed in your urine, feces, skin oils or hair growth. Another article says your fat is used as a place to store the toxic chemicals created in response to your negative feelings. If your body has a lot of toxins to store, your fat may be needed as a warehouse.

You know that if you eat more calories than you burn, your body will store the excess calories in your fat to be burned later in case you have the need. If you never get around to needing those calories stored in fat, your body is just going to hold on to them. You might think of your fat as "a thing", but it seems that your body recycles it and the stuff stored in it on an ongoing basis. If you change what you are eating, drinking, and thinking, your body might not need to hold onto your fat so that it has a place to keep your bad stuff.

121. Your Saliva pH Indicates the Stress of Your Thinking

By: Dr. Judith Giustini

Dr. M.T. Morter, MA, DC made this observation years ago: Stress causes changes in the pH of your saliva.

In Saliva pH Testing, which is performed 2 hours after you have had anything to eat, or anything to drink except water, test the pH of your saliva.

The challenge is: holding a Vitamin C tablet on your tongue for a few seconds, and removing it as soon as you can taste it. Then you swallow your saliva 4 times, and test your saliva pH again.

This test shows what your body does in response to the "threat" of the acid of the vitamin C.

The color of your pH paper in your original test will be yellow, green or blue. The color of your pH paper after your vitamin C challenge will be yellow, green or blue.

Where your saliva pH starts out and where it ends up indicates the degree of difficulty of your case. See 122 "Degree of Difficulty of Cases".

122. Degree of Difficulty of Cases

By: Dr. Judith Giustini

According to Dr. M. T. Morter, Jr., MA, DC, the pH of your saliva before and after you hold a vitamin C tablet on your tongue for a few seconds, indicates the degree of stress you are under, and this is an indicator as to the relative difficulty of your case. Where you start out will affect how long it will take for you to get results.

FIRST DEGREE - **Green to Blue**: Life may have handed you some strife, but your attitude is good. You handle stress well. Eliminate empty calories from your diet and choose organic foods.

SECOND DEGREE – **Yellow to Green or Blue**: Your body is on guard most of the time due to anxiety or stress. You doubt your worthiness. Avoid sugar, eat six servings of fruits and vegetables.

THIRD DEGREE - **Blue to Green or Green to Yellow**: You have been under low level stress due to worry for a long time. Your body is moving towards exhaustion. Your self-esteem is low. You need to remodel your belief system. Eat mostly fruits, vegetables and brown rice, with animal protein less than 40 grams per day.

FOURTH DEGREE - **Blue to Blue**: You are constantly seriously worried or anxious. You are tired a lot. You tend to feel like a victim and you may be blaming others for your problems. You need to acknowledge The Law of Cause and Effect. Add more raw vegetables to your diet.

FIFTH DEGREE - **Green to Green**: You are constantly dealing with strong emotions such as fear, anger or rage. You may feel like a martyr. You are heading for physical and emotional exhaustion. Decrease animal protein and add fruit and cooked vegetables.

SIXTH DEGREE - **Yellow to Yellow**: You are experiencing such strong emotions of hate, anger or rage that you may need medication for sleep. You are seriously ill. Your self-esteem is very low. Your diet should consist mostly of cooked vegetables.

123. Your Urinary pH

By: Dr. Judith Giustini

pH is a measurement of acidity or alkalinity, in this case, of your urine. The pH papers we use show pH from 5.5 (acid)to 8.0 (alkaline). Every food you eat leaves an acid or alkaline pH "ash" after it is burned in your body.

Your urinary pH reflects whether you have been consuming acid ash foods or alkaline ash foods. If you consume too many acid-ash foods, your urinary pH may paradoxically be alkaline, because you have created an emergency situation with too much acid, and your body needed to neutralize it with ammonia, which is very alkaline.

Foods that leave an acid ash are high protein foods, such as meats, poultry, fish, dairy products, eggs, beans and grains. Most fruits and vegetables leave an alkaline ash.

Your body was designed to run at a slightly alkaline pH. A good goal would be for you to consume 75% to 80% fruits and vegetables. See: *An Apple a Day, is it Enough Today?* by Dr. M.T. Morter, Jr., MA, DC

If the foods you eat are mostly acid, this can put your body in the "fight-or-flight" mode, where healing is not a priority. You can learn to test your urine pH at home, and understand the meaning of the results. Urine pH is an inexpensive scientific test that lets you keep track of how you are doing with your diet, and take charge of things in your life. See also: Ch. 127. What is Your Alkaline Reserve?

124. Is it Obesity or PTSD?

By: Dr. Judith Giustini

There are many causes of obesity, such as what you eat and drink, lack of exercise, etc., and what about all that emotional baggage? You may have many physical causes of your obesity, while at the same time being tormented by unresolved negative feelings buried alive in your subconscious mind. These negative feelings may be related to memories of adverse childhood (or later) experiences that you think you have already dealt with, but they are causing Post-Traumatic Stress Disorder and you don't know what they are, because they are subconscious.

If you have feelings such as unfulfilled or seeking love, you don't know why you feel motivated to consume more calories than you need, and the result will be overeating and overweight which cause you to feel like a victim and validate your low self-esteem.

If you are seriously trying to become a normal weight person and you keep sabotaging yourself, maybe it is time to find out what those buried feelings are and learn to forgive them.

125. Mind-Body Therapy vs. Obesity

By: Dr. Judith Giustini

If you are struggling with your weight, you are not alone. Just look around. Every day you spend in your fat body is a day of interference with your health, happiness, and success. To lose weight, you need to consume fewer calories than you burn. Unfortunately, there are many obstacles to accomplishing this. Maybe you get sabotaged by your habits, by the plethora of food and drink choices in pretty boxes, by fast food, by low blood sugar, by family and friends, by fears, suppressed love languages, PTSD, etc.

You are the person who is putting the food in your mouth. Why do you make the wrong choices? Maybe it's lack of knowledge. Maybe it's lack of self-control, but why? You are a very complicated person. It is important for you to know which causes are affecting you and in which priority they need to be dealt with. Maybe your obesity is being caused by chronic dehydration.

Obesity is an illness that is a cause of other illnesses. It can shorten your life on this planet and make you miserable while you are still here. Even though there are a lot of fat people around, there is still a lot of prejudice about obesity. Even if people don't say anything, they may still be thinking criticism your way.

In Mind-Body Therapy, we are looking for the thoughts, feelings, beliefs and memories that are behind it the causes of your obesity. This work can be done in person or remotely. It is not a substitute for a weight loss coach, but it will help you take charge of things in your life.

126. What is Your Alkaline Reserve?

By: Dr. Judith Giustini

In his *book An Apple a Day? Is it enough today?* Dr. M. Ted Morter, Jr, says that *our bodies are alkaline by design, but acid by function*, meaning that our cells function best in a sightly alkaline environment. Fruits and vegetables leave an alkaline ash after they are burned in your body. Animal foods leave a strongly acid ash, and other foods leave a more acid ash or less acid ash

Your cells make acid when you do anything – eating, breathing, golfing, worrying, etc. Your body is always getting rid of acid. The weak acids can be eliminated through your lungs, but the strong acids have to go out through your kidneys. Fruits and vegetables provide nutrients that help your body neutralize the acid of animal proteins. This is called your *alkaline reserve.*

Urine pH test: Using pH paper (range 5.5 – 8.0) Test pH of 1st morning urine, then go 2 days on diet of no fruits and no vegetables for 2 days. Test pH of first morning urine on 3rd day.

5.5 - 5.8 (yellow) means your alkaline reserve is adequate.

6.0 - 6.6 (green) means your alkaline reserve is running low.

6.8 - 8.0 (blue) means your alkaline reserve is zilch. Your urine may smell of ammonia.

Maybe you could try Super Shakes (Ch. 163) made with fruits and vegetables.

127. Gout, Arthritis and Diabetes

By: Dr. Judith Giustini

<u>Gout</u> is a painful, red and swollen condition that often occurs at the base of the big toe. It is so painful that the person can hardly stand the pressure of a bed sheet over it. Gout can also affect the ankles, wrists, knees and elbows. The cause of the pain is the accumulation of uric acid crystals in the joint. Uric acid forms from purine, which is a product of incomplete digestion of meat and fish. Uric acid crystals are very sharp, and they irritate the joint and surrounding tissues.

<u>Osteoarthritis</u> is a degenerative joint disease that affects about 20% of older people in the U.S. It usually develops in the fingers, knees, and hips and causes many missed days of work.

<u>Rheumatoid Arthritis</u> is an autoimmune disorder that affects the hands and feet, where the joints may become disfigured and require replacement.

In **<u>Type 2 diabetes,</u>** blood tests show high blood sugar and relative lack of insulin. It often affects obese people and may cause heart attack, stroke and/or blindness.

What these conditions have in common is that they usually occur in persons who have been eating too much animal protein (especially meat) for too long, which results in acidosis, which can be seen on a urine pH test. Try: a diet of strictly vegetables until your urine pH becomes normal.

Chronic dehydration is another main cause of these conditions.

Remedy: 64+ oz. water per day.

128. How Much Protein Do You Need?

By: Dr. Judith Giustini

Protein is important. Protein is a major component in your75 trillion cells. Your DNA and your hair are made of protein.

The U.S. government recommends 44-56 grams of protein per day for females, depending on age, and a little more for males, depending on age. Some authorities say 20-30 grams is adequate.

Chapter 224. in this book is "Your Urinary pH Indicates Your Dietary Stress". You can do this test yourself, if you get some pH paper that tests from 5.5 to 8.0 (amazon?). Chapter 235. in this book is "What is Your Alkaline Reserve? Your pH is of vital importance to your health, happiness and success. Too bad they don't teach this in junior high school.

Your body requires ample water each day to do the work it needs to do. Soda and beer are wet, but they are not water. If you have a high protein diet, and you are dehydrated, this is a ticket to high blood pressure, diabetes, heart attacks and strokes. If you drink at least 64 oz. of water per day. As you age, your perception of thirst becomes diminished. Patients at the dialysis clinic say they don't drink much water. If you are drinking enough water, your urine will be very light in color. If you are not overindulging in protein, there will be very few bubbles in the water.

129. Hypoglycemia

By: Dr. Judith Giustini

hypo = low, glyc = sugar, emia = blood.

Hypoglycemia is not a disease. It is a description of something your body is doing in response to your consuming too much sugar, white flour, or alcohol.

Your pancreas (Ch. 207. and 208.) has the job of releasing insulin in response to the amount of sugar in your blood stream. When your blood sugar becomes elevated to 120 or so, your pancreas normally secretes insulin, and your blood sugar returns to 70 or 80 within a couple of hours.

When you have hypoglycemia, your pancreas does not work right away in response to elevated blood sugar. Maybe it is overworked. By the time it does react, your blood sugar may be up to 170 or 180, which is an "emergency", and your pancreas secretes excess insulin, so your blood sugar goes way down, and you get cranky and irritable, or you get a headache or fall asleep. You crave sugar, and when you consume it, this starts the wild up and down blood sugar. Your medicine is your poison.

Eventually, your pancreas becomes exhausted and unable to respond to glucose in your blood, so your fasting blood sugar is elevated. You have diabetes. If you are dehydrated, and it is robbing water from your blood stream, this can show up as diabetes and high blood pressure.

130. Why Would You Need to Have a 5-Hour Glucose Tolerance Test?

By: Dr. Judith Giustini

According to *The Merck Manual*, your blood sugar should be between 70 (fasting) and 110 (after you eat a meal). Low levels of sugar in the blood (below 60) interfere with the functioning of many organ systems and your brain.

When your blood sugar is low, you might become cranky, snappish, irritable, testy, impatient or confused. You might get headaches or fall asleep in meetings or while driving your car. You may crave sweets or alcohol. You may gain weight. Friends may avoid you when you become "frantic".

Hypoglycemia is said to be "pre-diabetic". This can be because you have over-consumed refined sugar and your pancreas has become exhausted. It is important for you to know what your blood sugar does in response to a dose of glucose. The 5-Hour GTT is not a pleasant little test. It takes 5 hours, and you might not feel very well for the rest of the day after it, but it is important for you to know this information if you need to change your diet before you give yourself diabetes.

Your primary care doc may not understand why you want this test and may not order it for you. Maybe you can share this information with him or her.

A woman finally got her MD to prescribe a 2-Hour GTT. Her results were: Fasting: 97, 1 Hr.: 197, 2 Hr.: 157.If the test had gone on, there would likely have been a time when her blood sugar was quite low. She received a letter from her doctor, saying that the results of her test were "Normal".

131. Eating Toxic Foods: Pork, Shellfish, Scavengers

By: Dr. Judith Giustini

In The Bible at Leviticus Ch. 11. God was speaking to Moses and Aaron. and he gave a list of the foods that His people should not eat because they are not good for you, such as:

The camel, the rock badger, the hare and the pig. About pigs, He said you should not even touch their dead body because they are unclean.

Fish that have fins and scales are okay. This excludes shellfish and catfish.

Avoid eating: the eagle, the osprey, the vulture, the raven, the osprey, the gull, the swan, the pelican, and the bat.

1 Timothy 4:1-4 says you can eat *"all the foods which God created to be partaken of",* so, not the ones listed above. This is for your benefit because they are not good for you.

Being on a low-calorie diet is a struggle. You have to be on it from millisecond to millisecond. It's like penance. You did this to yourself - maybe due to Confusion, ignorance or self-indulgence and now you are paying your dues. This is great! You are coming to Self-Awareness Self-Knowledge, and taking charge of things in your life.

There's life after a pork roast dinner and a lobster salad sandwich. If you love yourself, why do you want to make yourself sick?

132. Overeating (Why?)

By: Dr. Judith Giustini

In her book *Feelings Buried Alive Never Die,* Karol K. Truman lists some possible feelings causing "***Over-Eating*** (Compulsive)" as: "Tension, feeling a material-emotional lack, craving closeness, putting on emotional armor, A symbol of power and a desire to throw ones' weight around".

Your body can only use about 2,000 calories per day if you are a normal-weight woman, and 2,500 if you are a normal-weight man. If you give your body more than it needs at the moment, your body keeps it around for when you might need it. Maybe you don't pig-out – just a couple of hundred extra calories here, and a couple of hundred extra calories there. 1 Tbs. of butter is 100 calories. Some breakfast items at the drive-thru are 1,000 calories. How many calories are in that bedtime snack of chocolate ice cream or in those couple of glasses of wine? You need Calorie Consciousness (Ch160.) and Nutritional Awareness (Ch. 161.)

Maybe you have been on a diet that is high in calories, but low in nutrients- pasta, pizza, donuts, ice cream burgers, fries, etc., Your body will be looking for "real" nutrients, such as those found in fruits and vegetables. But lacking those items in your diet, it may turn to consuming additional amounts of those empty-calorie foods, since those are the ones, you are making available. Your body is starving for food, and you are giving it junk. Your body has a dandy place to store those extra calories – right in your belly fat and your pudgy rear end. If you choose to become a normal-weight person, you are going to have to make a decision that you are ready to do what it takes and take charge of things in your life.

133. How Much Food Do You Need to Eat to Feel Satisfied?

By: Dr. Judith Giustini

A pudgy woman in her 60's took insulin for her diabetes. For work, he took care of children in her home – usually one child at a time. One reason she liked to work from home was so that she would be near her kitchen, because she had a strong attachment to food, going back to her childhood when she often went to bed hungry. She said she had tried to lose weight, but she needed a to feel a certain degree of fullness in her stomach to feel satisfied, so she remained fat.

A few years ago, there were "fat shows" on TV. On these shows, morbidly obese people would go to a camp, where they would eat less and exercise more. Some of the people complained about the size of food portions, which were actually quite large.

Some people would not feel satisfied on a diet that only allows small portions, but foods vary widely in the number of calories they contain. One cup of green beans is about 30 calories and one cup of ice cream is about 300 calories.

In the program of a very successful weight loss group, most vegetables are unlimited, so you don't have to count the calories and you can eat as much as you want. You can learn some low-calorie toppings for your vegetables to make them seem tasty to you. Vegetables are full of nutrients in a highly absorbable form, so eating them is good for your health. On some diets, you don't have to count the calories of apples, hard-boiled eggs or skinless chicken breast.

134. Thyroid Malfunction Due to Stress

By: Dr. Judith Giustini

From Google: The thyroid gland is a butterfly-shaped gland in the front of your neck under your skin. It is part of your endocrine system and controls many of your body's important functions by producing and secreting hormones. (FYI: There is a great article on Wikipedia.)

Hypothyroidism due to insufficient production of thyroid hormones, which may be related to lack of iodine in diet or other causes. Symptoms: abnormal weight gain, constipation, cold intolerance and slow heart rate.

Hyperthyroidism due to excess production of thyroid hormones. Symptoms: Weight loss, excessive appetite.

In her book *Feelings Buried Alive Never Die,* Karol K. Truman lists some feelings that may be hidden causes of your thyroid malfunction:

- Conflict between the conscious & the subconscious
- Lack of love for Self
- Fears self-expression
- Deep sense of frustration/anxiety
- Lack of discernment

In Mind-Body Therapy, we are looking to understand you. Maybe you have negative feelings due adverse childhood (or other) experiences buried alive in your subconscious mind. We can find out. Your MD can prescribe testing for your thyroid and give you medication if you need it. If you still have the problem, maybe we need to do a Search.

135. Chronic Stress of Self-Loathing Due to Obesity

By: Dr. Judith Giustini

You know what it's like. Those darn sneaky pounds. You thought you were being careful with your diet, but somehow you gained a pound last month. Fat is not fun. It's those jiggles in your backside with every step. It's that girth around your middle. . . Maybe you have been on a series of diets over the years, and after you lose all your weight and buy a new wardrobe, those pesky pounds sneak back on your body. You are frustrated, hatin' on yourself, reluctant to try again, especially after all that time you spent depriving yourself. Maybe you are confused, can't focus, plus you have other things to worry about.

Food is a big subject – lots of science. Maybe you can study and develop Nutritional Awareness, but what about just starting with Calorie Consciousness, since that's a major key to dieting success.

In Mind-Body Therapy, you go from Confusion (Yakin' & Crankin') to Clarity (That was then, this is now.) to Self-Knowledge (There's life after), and maybe even to Peace. Negative feelings buried in your subconscious mind have power over you, even if you don't know what they are. They affect the way your trillions of cells function.

In her book *Feelings Buried Alive Never Die,* Karol K. Truman says that one of the feelings associated with **Overweight** is Unexpressed, mis-perceived & inappropriate feelings. One such feeling is **Unforgiveness,** and the feeling that energetically neutralizes it is **I am Accepting**.

In Mind-Body Therapy, you can find out which feelings are affecting you and take charge of them through Forgiveness (winning by letting go).

136. Subconscious Causes of Stress

By: Dr. Judith Giustini

When you are not feeling well, you tend to focus on what is going wrong with your body and what you don't like and worrying about what's going to happen if things get worse.

What you think about you bring about; what you see (visualize with feelings) is what you get; what you fear comes near. When you focus on what is wrong, you are going to attract more of what is wrong. What you eat, drink, and breathe and how you exercise and rest are habit patterns linked into your belief system. Your choices in these areas have a profound effect on your health, happiness, and success.

What negative feelings are running and running like an old movie in your subconscious mind? Is it something you did that you regret? Is it something somebody did to you that you have not forgiven? Are you enslaved to your mortgage or credit card debts? Subconscious negative feelings can cause chronic stress that can overwhelm every system in your body.

There is a program in your subconscious mind that directs the activities of every cell, tissue and organ in your body. The subconscious Power That Runs Your Body is supposed to be interactive with The Power That Made Your Body throughout your life, but stress can interfere with this subconscious relationship.

You can forgive the negative feelings that are causing your stress and replace them with the positive feelings that energetically neutralize them. This will take away their power over you, and you will be winning by letting go.

137. Overeating, which Causes Excess Nutrients to be Stored as Fat

By: Dr. Judith Giustini

Maybe you went to an All-You Can Eat Buffet and you "pigged-out", or it was a holiday at Grandma's and you "just had to" sample all the dishes. After you eat anything, it gets digested in your stomach and small intestine, and the nutrients are picked up into your bloodstream and sent to your liver for more processing, and later they sent to all of your trillions of cells so they can do their job of keeping you alive.

There is only "so much" of whatever you ate that can be of use to your cells at any given time, so your body stores the excess nutrients as fat. Here's more news: whenever you consume 3,500 calories more than you burn, you gain 1 lb., even if that's just a few calories here and a few calories there.

An adult female of "normal" weight can consume about 2,000 calories per day without gaining or losing weight. For an adult male, it's 2,500. When you are obese, it takes more calories to move the mass over the distance, so that number can be higher when your weight is higher. After you lose weight, you will no longer be able to consume the same quantity of food without gaining weight.

If you are going to lose those extra lbs., you are going to need a plan. A time-honored weight loss formula is 1,200 calories per day for a woman and 1,500 calories per day for a man. You need to stick to this diet day in and day out, millisecond to millisecond to reach your goal weight. (Ch. 162. Super Soup, 163. Super Shakes,165. Stir-Fry). On this program, you will lose about 2 lbs. per week. You need to develop Calorie Consciousness (Ch. 160.)

138. Frustration Due to Physical Limitations Caused by Obesity

By: Dr. Judith Giustini

Maybe you used to be fit and trim back I the day when you were a cheerleader for the high school, the captain of the basketball team, or active in military service. But then the kids came along, the job was sedentary, you had a long drive to and from work, you were very busy, so you frequently opted for meals from the drive-thru window. Maybe you got he "COVID-19" (pounds you gained during the Pandemic. Maybe carrying around those extra lbs. has caused you to need a knee replacement or a hip replacement. Maybe it's too embarrassing for you to appear in a swimsuit or in tights at the YMCA.

Maybe you have tried to lose weight by skipping meals or by going on a fast, only to be defeated by hunger. Maybe you "rewarded" your poor, deprived self by indulging in your favorite treats. Maybe it's annoying sitting home with your physical limitations while your friends are out golfing or hiking in the Adirondacks, so maybe you go to the store and park in the Handicapped spot and buy yourself a few treats. Tomorrow. maybe you'll regret it and nibble some treats to make you feel better.

If you choose to become a normal-weight person, you can't keep doing what you have been doing and expect a different result. You need a Plan. If your main problem is lack of knowledge, you need to develop Calorie Consciousness (Ch. 160} and Nutritional Awareness (Ch. 161.). If you are going to reach your goal weight, you might have to be on a diet for a long time, while losing 2 lbs./week. Cheer up. On a plant-based diet, you can stuff yourself on "allowed" foods and keep on losing weight. You can set yourself free.

139. Stuck in a Situation – Kids, Job, etc.

By: Dr. Judith Giustini

Maybe you are at home, doing childcare and housewife stuff. or working outside the home, and still doing all those household duties, and it's just so difficult to focus on your diet. Maybe you are a Dad, and, with your work and family life, you don't get to the YMCA on a regular basis, so you are developing a "Dad Bod".

Everybody's life is different, but a calorie is still a calorie and itis so difficult to get rid of those extra lbs. once they come to inhabit your once-svelte body, so you buy bigger clothes.

Maybe now is the time for you to learn some health and nutrition facts. If you are a normal-weight woman, you will gain weight if you consume more than 2,000 calories per day. For a normal-weight man, it's 2,500. If you choose not to be a behemoth, you need to develop Calorie Consciousness (Ch. 160.) and practice Defensive Dining (Ch. 37.) before you nibble your way to diabetes and go blind due to hardening of the arteries or have your leg amputated below the knee.

Take a look at how many calories are in pizza and fast foods. Most of the restaurant chains provide the calorie information about their menu items online. But even if you know how many calories they contain, that still does not make them good for you. You can get a USDA calorie chart online or order a book from amazon. If you can take charge of this very important facet of your life and live in a normal-weight body, you will be in much better health, and you will be setting a good example for your friends and relations

140. Feeling Deprived of Favorite Foods Due to Diet

By: Dr. Judith Giustini

In Ch. 117. "Why is it So Difficult to Change Your Habits?", it says, "What you eat and drink may *seem* to be <u>conscious</u> choices, but they are actually determined by programming in your subconscious mind that has become part of your belief system." They may have been influenced by your culture, by the foods and drinks you experienced in childhood, maybe even by your mother's choices of food and drink while she was pregnant to you, maybe even attached to memories of feelings from back then.

Your Belief System is like a stern "Parent". It is in charge of your "Shoulds" and "Oughts'". In addition to this programming, you have the food preferences you have developed in response to what has been available and convenient, to the point where you no longer have to read the menu to decide what you are going to order at the fast-food window. These are your Habits.

If what you have been eating and drinking has ended up with multiple pounds to lose, you are going to have to battle this tough opponent of your habits backed up by your belief system.

If you overeat by 100 calories per day for 35 days, you will gain 1 lb. A Big Mac is about 550 calories. A medium order of fries is about 350 calories. A 12-ounce soda is 150 calories.

It's easy to become all resolute about losing those extra lbs. after a big dinner when your tummy is full, but when it comes time to order a different burger choice, skip the fries, and order a smaller soda, maybe you will feel deprived, and Mr. Habits and Mr. Belief System will win again. How about if you skip the window and do something else?

141. Ongoing Struggle with Weight due to Confusion

By: Dr. Judith Giustini

Maybe you gained weight due to being "too busy" to shop for groceries and prepare wholesome meals for yourself. This was the excuse of a woman in Rhode Island who worked as the office manager for a group of about 10 lawyers. At the time, the lawyer business was kind of slow, and she was afraid of losing her job after 23 years, so she opted to eat 3 meals per day from the drive-thru. Unfortunately, she did not have Calorie Consciousness, and she was getting fat and kind of cranky, so, maybe they were looking for an excuse to cut her loose.

But she had other things on her mind – negative feelings that she was suppressing into her subconscious because they were so painful and embarrassing. But suppressing them just gave them more power over her. She also had a worsening problem with her ankles that caused her to be unsteady on her feet.

She was one of 8 children of her parents, all of whom that father had chosen to molest. In one incident, her father was in the back yard lying on a chaise in the sunshine and he asked her to bring him an iced tea. When she brought it, he also insisted that she give him blow -ob. After she moved into her own apartment, her father used visit her and demand sex, saying that if she did not do it with him, he would go home and molest her youngest brother. Somehow, a social worker found out about this, and her father moved to California with his wife and their younger children before he got in trouble.

This lady did not "get it" about subconscious emotional stress as a possible cause of her symptoms and she went back to her Chiropractor to get an adjustment.

142. Irritation by Crazy-Making People Causes Nibbling

By: Dr. Judith Giustini

A very fat 55-year-old woman from North Attleboro, MA was living at home with her parents, who were schoolteachers getting ready to retire. She had moved home about 16 years earlier to help her parents. She did the chores, the landscaping, the bookkeeping, the grocery shopping and the meal preparation.

Starting in childhood, this woman had a contentious relationship with her mom. The lady next door said she remembered hearing them screaming at one another in the summer when the windows were open years ago. Seems her mom favored her 2 sons, and her2 daughters got shortchanged. After her dad died and it was just the daughter and the mother (who, by now, sinking into dementia) and there was a lot of bickering, and the homemade cookies were close at hand, as were the Hallowe'en candies and the leftover goodies from the MLM meeting in her parlor, so she did a lot of mindless nibbling.

The daughter also had baggage from a failed boyfriend relationship where she was duped into thinking she was the only lady staying over at his place certain nights per week (but nope, he also had another girlfriend.

The irritation of dealing with her crazy-making mother, plus the sadness of being duped by her boyfriend, kept Calorie Consciousness far away from her mind. In her book *Feelings Buried Alive Never Die,* Karol K. Truman says that **Obesity** is connected with "A feeling of power and a desire to throw one's weight around".

143. Lack of Minerals Drives You to Eat More

By: Dr. Judith Giustini

In our country, we have many large commercial farms that use science-based fertilizers to get a good crop. Still, our soils are known to be depleted of certain minerals that should be in our food. Refined foods, donuts, chips, soda, etc. lack minerals. Fresh raw fruits and vegetables contain minerals in a usable form, plus, they contain enzymes that help them to be digested in your system. Cooked fruits and vegetables contain minerals, but no enzymes. Meats, fish, dairy products and eggs are sources for minerals in a usable form, plus proteins. If you are on a mostly plant-based diet that includes eggs and milk for protein, you may need to take an iron supplement and an iodine supplement.

Everything you eat and drink needs to be digested. Enzymes and digestive juices are made from the nutrients in your diet. But your body can't make minerals. They need to be supplied in your diet. When your body is lacking in minerals, it may impel you consume food, looking for them. If you interpret this urge as "hunger", you may just reach for something to fill up your stomach, and if you choose to give it junk food, it will have something else to digest, and you will become more nutritionally deficient. plus, you will have added however many calories and calories DO count.

Fruits and vegetables contain minerals in a form that your body can readily use them, but how can you conveniently include them in your diet? How about Super Soup (Ch. 162), Super Shakes (Ch. 163) and Stir-Frys (Ch. 165.)? If you try it for a week, you may notice that you are not venously hungry, and you have more cash in your pocket. See also: Are You Addicted to Empty Calories? (Ch. 11), Beware Fragmented Foods (Ch. 17.), Minerals are Essential for Your Health (Ch. 70.), and Signs of Mineral Deficiency (Ch. 82.)

144. Additional Food - Requires Additional Nutrients

By: Dr. Judith Giustini

Whatever food, beverage or substance you swallow requires your body to deal with it. Maybe that's via digestion, processing through your liver, eliminated through your lungs, kidneys or intestine. If it is not digested or adequately processed, it can become a poison. Since your body's main job is to keep you alive, it has systems and backup systems to do this job, even if it must rob minerals from your bones to get its work done. Some signs of mineral deficiency are flabby skin, weak muscles, poor digestion, lethargy and lowered immunity. (See AOO 82. Signs of Mineral Deficiency.)

It is a big and constant job for your body to deal with everything you ingest, it needs specific chemicals to go in saliva, stomach acid, pancreatic enzymes, liver bile, etc. Where does it get the ingredients for these products? It gets them from your diet. If you are consuming a diet of fragmented foods, chips. and soda, it is not going to have the proper chemicals to deal with more complex molecules, and you may find yourself staying away from foods that are too difficult to digest, which means fewer nutrients to keep your trillions of cells functioning properly, and you may find that certain foods "don't agree" with you, or you get the sour burps and you "need to" to take an antacid or maybe you get diarrhea.

Antacids cause an "emergency" in your body by making your stomach super alkaline, so your body is forced to respond by producing extra acid to deal with the emergency, and your body can use the acid to digest whatever it is that you put in your stomach. Your body needs the vitamins, minerals, and enzymes of whole foods to do its job of keeping you alive.

145. Additional Food Contributes to Weight Gain

By: Dr. Judith Giustini

"So", you may say, "everybody knows that.", and you would be right, but maybe we could dig a little deeper and see some of the "why's", in case this applies to you. In AOO11. Are You Addicted to Empty Calories? it says, Empty calories are made up of small molecules that digest rapidly. If you have been living on a diet ow white bread, pasta, sugar and alcohol, your body may not have the ability to digest large molecules. You may seem to be addicted to empty calorie foods because they may be all you are able to digest. This type of diet causes "Reactive Hypoglycemia" (Ch. 131.), where your blood sugar spikes way up in reaction to you ate something sugary, then plummets way down, maybe depriving your brain of nutrition, and you are driven to eat something else sweet to get your blood sugar out of the basement. When this scenario is repeated over and over, it can lead to adrenal exhaustion, and your get-up-and-go will have got-up-and-gone. Did I mention nutritional deficiencies? You may be gaining weight, but your cells are starving. Soon won't be able to work properly leading to downward-mobile with your health (and what will that do to your happiness and success?)

In her book *Feelings Buried Alive Never Die,* Karol K Truman says that some people who have ***Over-Eating*** (Compulsive)" are operating according to a program described as "Emotional energy based on anger and resentment". If that's you, why is that?

Ch.84. is "Some Ways Sugar Ruins Your Health". Ch. 19. is "Carbohydrates". Ch. 20. is "Carbohydrates Are Not Evil". There is a way out, but you have to be ready to Divorce Your Old Diet (Ch. 41.) So go ahead and check out the recipe for Super Shakes (Ch. 163.) and learn about Calorie Consciousness) Ch. 160.) and Nutritional Awareness (Ch. 161.)

146. Poor Digestion Due to Lack of Digestants

By: Dr. Judith Giustini

Maybe you were on a poor diet in the past. You thought you were eating what you liked because you liked what you were eating. There can be many motivations and influences on your choices of food and drink, but maybe you are having the sour burps or your bowels are not doing a good job. How can you take better care of yourself?

If your poor diet has left your body without the chemicals it needs to build your stomach acid you need, cheer up. You can get a product such as Betaine Hydrochloride with Pepsin for $17 or so for 250 tabs. on amazon. If you need pancreatic enzymes, you can get those as well for $19.97 for 60. These could be a crutch for you when you are starting out on a whole foods diet. Maybe your MD can advise you about dosage, but you can also do your own research and see what works for you.

Every step of your digestive process requires water – for your saliva, for your stomach juices, for the liquid that comes from your pancreas to bring enzymes to your small intestine, for the blood that transports your digested foods to your liver, for the arterial blood that transports food and oxygen to every cell in your body for the venous blood" . . . for lymphatic fluid, elimination, etc. Also, your brain is a big user of water. "Authorities" recommend from 64 oz. per day to ½ ounce for every lb. you weigh. Chronic dehydration has been linked to high blood pressure, diabetes, heart attacks and strokes.

In her book *Feelings Buried Alive Never Die*, among the causes of *"Indigestion"*, she lists feelings such as: "Feeling everyone is against you, feel you need to fight your way through life, Feelings of anxiety, and Fear of losing job, losing security" as *"Probable Feelings Causing Illness"*. What/who do you need to Forgive?

147. Antacid Drugs Require the Body to Supply More Acid

By: Dr. Judith Giustini

When you have the sour burps, and you (correctly) get the idea that your food is not digesting as it should, maybe you will opt for an antacid drug, such as those advertised on TV. So, you take the drug, and yep! the sour burps ae over and your food seems to have digested, so you guess the drug has worked.

But no, your digestive system worked because you created an emergency. Your body makes the hydrochloric acid that your stomach uses to digest your food. If your food is not digesting, it is not because your stomach needs to become more alkaline because you took an antacid drug. When you take an antacid drug, you make your stomach more alkaline and less able to digest your food, so now there is an emergency, and your body has to respond, because the undigested food could become a poison and kill you. So now your body goes into emergency mode and does whatever it has to do to gather up the chemicals – maybe from other places in your body where they are also scarce, thus interfering with something else your body is working on.

Your body is a very sophisticated chemical factory. It needs certain raw materials that come from fruits and vegetables to do its work. The old adage, "You are what you eat" might more appropriately be, "You are what you eat, and your body can digest and process into nutrients your body can make into those things that become *you*".

Eating more fruits and vegetables can seem like a daunting task. It is so much easier to just get something fast at the drive-thru window, but not if you have a blender. (Ch. 163.)

Poor digestion can be your ticket to premature aging and all the medical consequences that come with that. Nursing home, anybody?

148. Diarrhea Due to Inability to Digest Foods

By: Dr. Judith Giustini

Your digestive system is aware of the foods you consume on a regular basis, and it does the best it can with the chemical tools you provide it to work with to break these foods into the nutrients it needs to keep you alive. But maybe you go to an ethnic restaurant, and you order up some dishes that contain things your body does not have the tools to process, so it mobilizes its resources to get this strange stuff out of you before it can turn into a poison. If you are looking to add new foods to your diet, you may have to introduce them slowly, in small quantities.

But what if your digestive system is "not playing with a full deck", due to dehydration or lack of nutrients to provide the raw materials your body needs to build your stomach acid, your pancreatic enzymes and your liver bile. There may be a lot of foods your body is unable to cope with, which gives it a reason to get rid of them fast. If you are also dehydrated, this is going complicate the problem, and your body may need to borrow water from your blood stream to deal with the emergency, thus increasing your overall dehydration.

In his book *Diabetes, Cancer, Depression – Their Common Cause and Natural Cure,* Dr. F. Batmanghelidj says, "preventing dehydration prevents serious diseases". He says that your brain functions on the energy from water, and that drinking enough water can restore your enthusiasm and fill you with the joys of life. He says that some dehydrated persons have lost 30 to 50 lbs. just by drinking enough water daily. He says that water is a natural anti-cancer medication.

You will have to discipline yourself to drink the proper amount of water... See Ch. 117. Why is it So Difficult to Change Your Habits?

149. Poor Digestion Due to Dehydration

By: Dr. Judith Giustini

Water is necessary for every step of digestion. Water is a major component of your saliva, your stomach acids, the fluid from your pancreas that brings digestive enzymes to your small intestine, the bile from your liver that is stored in your gall bladder, the blood in your arteries that picks up nutrients from your small intestine and carries it to your liver, then transports it from your liver to each and every one of your trillions of cells, and in the fluid in your lymphatic system that deals with cellular wastes. Water is needed to move your digesting food through your small intestine and the waste into and through your colon, where your body harvests water from the waste before passing the waste out of your body.

Water is not an expensive pharmaceutical drug. It is pretty available to everybody in most places in the world, so why are some people suffering from heartburn and indigestion due to chronic dehydration? What you Drink can be affected by What you Think– maybe not your conscious thoughts, because it is your belief system that is like a stern "Parent" that is in charge of your "shoulds and oughts" and you don't even think about questioning it. But if you are having indigestion or heartburn, maybe your body is trying to tell you something.

How much water do you drink on a daily basis? What other symptoms of dehydration do you have – constipation? allergies? high blood pressure? diabetes? obesity? migraines? low back pain? Once you "know" that you may be causing some of your health problems by not drinking enough water, why is it so difficult to just start in "doing it right" from there on out? It is difficult to change your habits. You have to discipline yourself to drink those 64 oz. of water each day.

150. Constipation Due to Dehydration

By: Dr. Judith Giustini

In his book *You're Not Sick, You're Thirsty!* Dr. F. Batmanghelidj tells us that when you are dehydrated, your body goes into "drought management", trying to save the precious water for places where it is vitally needed. After your food is digested in your stomach and small intestine, the residue goes to your large intestine for elimination.

When you are dehydrated, your body slows down the elimination of your feces so it can salvage as much water as it can before it has to let go of this stash of water. This causes your feces to become hard, with not fluid enough to flow. Dr. Batmanghelidj says that chronic dehydration can lead to cancer formation in the large intestine and the rectum". It can also cause a painful situation in the lower abdomen that mimics the symptoms of appendicitis.

Some cases of constipation have required medical treatment such as having to have a doctor or a nurse remove the feces manually by picking it out of the anus. At a salon of colonic irrigation in Massachusetts, a man called on Saturday for an emergency visit. The therapist weighed him before his colonic irrigation and after it, and he had lost 8 lbs.

Another patient was a woman suffering from pollen allergies. She was having daily bowel movements, but her colonics were full of feces – maybe it had been stuck to the walls of her colon? This went on for 40 sessions until one day it happened that there was something so large that it could not pass through the tube of the machine, so she sat on the toilet, and she was able to force a large ball of feces out of her rectum. After that, there was hardly any fecal matter in the water of the colonic machine, and her allergies were a no more.

151. Elevated Blood Cholesterol Due to Dehydration

By: Dr. Judith Giustini

In his book *You're Not Sick, You're Thirsty!* Dr. F. Batmanghelidj devotes several pages to this topic. He said that when you are dehydrated, your body uses cholesterol as a protective "clay" covering in areas such as your liver and the lining of your arteries that come in contact with the blood laden with digested food after it leaves your liver small intestine.

When this concentrated blood reaches your brain, and your brain realizes you are dehydrated, it signals you to become thirsty, so you drink water, but by then the cholesterol protective response has already occurred. In chronic dehydration, additional amounts of cholesterol will be produced by your liver cells, and your body will use as sort of a "protective clay" in your liver and arteries to prevent the water from their cells being osmotically transferred to dilute the concentration of the blood.

"To prevent excess cholesterol deposits in the cells lining the arteries and the liver, you need to drink regularly an ample amount of water a half hour before food intake. By this action, the cells of the body will become well hydrated before confronting the concentrated blood after food intake." He recommends drinking 2 glasses of water ½ hour before you consume food to give your body time to become hydrated. In another part of the book, he advises drinking ½ ounce of water per day for every lb. you weigh, plus 1 tsp. of sea salt per gallon of water. (If you are very heavy, this could be quite a lot of water. Can you do 64 oz?

After a period of regulating daily water intake so that the cells become fully hydrated, the cholesterol defense system may be required less and its production and cholesterol will decrease.

152. Nutritional Content of Eggs From Internet research By: Dr. Judith Giustini

By: Dr. Judith Giustini

Per USDA: A large egg contains 78 calories, 5 g of Fat, 6 grams of Protein, 0.6 g of Carbohydrates, 62 mg. of Sodium, 147 mg. Choline, 0.5 g Sugars, and 0g Fibers. and many micronutrients.

Nutrition Facts – from a n article by Malia Frey, M.A., ACE-CHC, CPT, updated 2024

<u>Egg Health Benefits</u>

- The protein in eggs helps maintain muscle mass.
- The fats in eggs do not raise blood cholesterol.
- Nutrients in eggs protect eyes from macular. degeneration. 1 egg/20,000 contains Salmonella bacteria, which cause diarrhea and vomiting, if you eat it raw.
- Choline in eggs supports brain health vs. memory loss.

<u>Egg Varieties</u>

- There is no nutritional difference in brown/white eggs.
- Free Range: chickens can roam indoors and outdoors.

Cage Free: Chickens can roam indoors, perch and nest. Many people are allergic to eggs, so read food labels

<u>Adverse Effects</u>

1 egg/20,000 contains the Salmonella bacteria. Symptoms of Salmonella infection: diarrhea, fever, and stomach and abdominal cramps. Out of millions of salmonella infections per year, only about 420 deaths. "Pasteurized" eggs are safe to eat raw. The cholesterol in eggs is not seen to be a cause of elevated blood cholesterol.

153. Panic Due to Going to Bed Hungry

By: Dr. Judith Giustini

A woman in Rhode Island gained about 120 lbs. after she was injured on her job working for the office that tracks dead-beat Dads. Seems that when she left the area where she and the other workers had their desks, and came back in, somebody had carelessly left a wheelie desk chair in her path. She fell on it, and it scooted across the room and crashed into a desk, where she fell on the floor and injured her back.

She was home for quite a while after this, and she started gaining weight because she was nibbling cookies and treats. She had issues with men, so when her boyfriend would say anything about what she was eating, she would eat more for spite.

When she was young, her father abandoned her and her 5 siblings, and her mother had to work 2 cleaning jobs to support them. Sometimes, there wasn't enough food, and she would go to bed hungry. As an adult, it brought back bad memories if she went to bed hungry, so she made sure not to do that anymore.

It is quite possible to be on a low-calorie diet and not have to go to bed hungry. It takes planning. But she was upset about her workplace injury, and she couldn't focus on her diet. Her breakfast coffee was 250 calories, and she did not want to give it up.

When she was in school, she had fallen several times and injured her knees. Both of them needed replacing, the left one worse than the right. Her new bodyweight of 285 lbs. was making it difficult for her even to walk around. She "thought" she was angry at her husband for abandoning her and their 4 sons, but she was actually angry at her Dad, and she blamed him for making her go to bed hungry.

154. Trying to Diet While Doing Starvation in the Midst of Plenty

By: Dr. Judith Giustini

If you are obese, chances are that you did not gain all this weight on a diet 75 to 80% fruits and vegetables (fresh and raw preferrable because they contain enzymes to help your body digest them) and 20-25% everything else.

If you are trying to stay on a weight loss diet of 1,200 to 1,500 calories per day, there aren't many choices at the drive-thru window that are going to work for you. A Big Mac is about 550 calories, and a medium order of fries is about 350 calories. A large chocolate shake is 800 calories. You can have defeated you diet for the day by the time you put the paper wrappers back in the bag. Fast food supplies a lot of calories, but it lacks the nutrients you would be getting on a plant-based diet, so your cells are actually starving for nutrients, and you are giving them food that does not fulfill their needs, so they are actually starving.

If you choose to lose your excess bodyweight, you are going to need to commit toa different diet. If you go right back to your old "friendly" diet of fast foods after you reach your goal weight, you will be involved in the yo-yo weight syndrome (Ch. 94.), and this is very discouraging, like if you quit smoking (which is difficult to do) and you start smoking again, you will have to quit again or just give up trying. Smoking is bad for you and so is a low-nutrient diet.

When you are obese, you may have many negative feelings towards yourself because of your obesity, and many predisposing factors, going back to your childhood. Hopefully, this book will help you to understand yourself better. Maybe you would benefit from the help of a diet coach or some Mind-Body Therapy sessions.

155. Adrenal Exhaustion Due to the Stresses of Life/Emotions

By: Dr. Judith Giustini

Your adrenal glands sit atop your kidneys. They produce adrenaline in response to stress. Adrenaline is a hormone that quickly gets you body ready if you have to fight a bear or run away from a bear in the woods. After the emergency is over your adrenal glands are supposed to go back to their resting mode, to get ready for the next emergency.

Your negative feelings can be causes of stress. Emotions such as fear, hate and anger require adrenaline. According to research, it takes 72 hours for your body to get back to normal after you're getting angry once. But what if the emergency never stops? What if you are angry at yourself because of those extra lbs. you are being forced (because of who, what, when, where, why and how?) to be aware of them millisecond-to-millisecond day after day and night after night. After a while, your glands and organs are liable to fault-out.

In her book *Feelings Buried Alive Never Die,* Karol K. Truman says that certain illnesses are causally related to certain negative feelings. Under ***Adrenal Problems,*** she lists some "Probable feelings causing illness" as: Feels like a victim, no belief in self, "Don't care what happens to me" attitude, Lack of courage, Feelings of anxiety, Misusing the will, Subconscious belief that life must have burdens, Being disloyal to *self,* Unresolved jealousies & fears. and feels that one must struggle for success, power or position. These negative feelings keep running and running, like an old movie on an endless loop, attracting illness and life circumstances you do not like, and you don't know why.

156. Chronic Fatigue Makes You Worry About Yourself

By: Dr. Judith Giustini

Your Health Happiness and Success are largely dictated by: what you Eat, what you Drink, what you Breathe and how you Exercise, how you Rest and what you Think.

If you wake up tired in the morning after a full night of sleep, maybe you have coffee and a donut for breakfast, because these are quick to grab a the drive-up. Maybe your energy is okay for a while, but by mid-morning, you are fatigued and maybe cranky. If you have a sugary snack, it brings your energy up for a while, and then crashes back down because you have reactive hypoglycemia, or maybe you even have diabetes or some other health problems. Maybe you are dehydrated.

Maybe your Doc can run some tests and see if there's anything that can be treated medically. Sure, do that. You need to know this information and get all the help you can. According to The Law of Cause & Effect, your actions have Consequences. According to The Law of Attraction, what you think about you bring about, and What you fear comes near. Why did you attract obesity?

In her book *Feelings Buried Alive Never Die,* in the section ***Probable Feelings Causing Ill-ness***, under ***Chronic Fatigue Syndrome,*** she lists: "Feeling totally alone, Feelings of desolation, Feelings of despair, Feeling hopeless / "It's no use", Tired of trying to prove yourself, Low self-worth, and Has lost the will to live". Maybe you have one or some of these subconscious feelings, but which ones, why? Up-and-down energy and bouts of fatigue are symptoms not to be ignored. What is causing your symptoms?

157. Aches and Pains Due to Changing Diet too Fast

By: Dr. Judith Giustini

If you have been on a diet of pizza, pasta, chicken nuggets, burgers, etc., and your weight has been creeping up, maybe you had an "ah-ha!" moment and you decided to do something about it, like change to a vegetarian diet, but then you developed aches and pains, and you started having doubts about getting your weight under control, if this meant living with all this discomfort.

Fruits and vegetables leave an "alkaline ash" after they are burned (metabolized) in your body. Proteins, grains, etc., leave an "acid ash" If your body has been operating on a mostly acid-ash diet, and you suddenly get "Nutrition Religion", you may go through a period of aches and pains if you don't know that this is a common experience of persons making this radical change too quickly. See; AOO127. "What is Your Alkaline Reserve?" You can do the pH test described there.

Nany people carry 20-30 lbs. of toxic waste in their large intestine. Fruits and vegetables are cleansing. Maybe your body will be able to let go of some of this garbage, but it has to go through some processes for this, and you may experience some symptoms caused by this toxicity being in your bloodstream while it is being processed out of your body. This is a good time to be sure you are drinking the proper amount of water for yourself, to help with this cleanse. Maybe you could check into colonic irrigations.

In her book *Feelings Buried Alive Never Die*, Karol K. Truman lists as *"Probable Feelings Causing Ill-ness", under "Aches"*: "Feeling of being all alone, feeling separated from source of love, Feeling that nobody loves me, *Aching* to be held and loved . . . "

158. Calorie Consciousness

By: Dr. Judith Giustini

A calorie (definition) "is the energy needed to raise 1 gram of water through 1-degree centigrade". (Huh?) Almost everything you eat or drink has calories. Some foods contain more calories per quantity than other foods.

How many calories per day does it take to maintain your bodyweight, without gaining or losing? That is about 2,000 for a woman and 2,500 for a man. It is higher for obese people because it takes more energy(calories) to move the mass over the distance.

If you consume 3,500 calories (cumulatively) more than you burn, you gain 1 lb. This is easy to do, considering that a Big Mac is 550 calories, a large chocolate shake is 800 calories, and a medium order of fries is 350 calories, and some breakfast sandwiches are over 1,000 calories.

A time-honored weight loss formula is 1,200 calories per day for a woman and 1,500 calories per day for a man. You don't have to be a victim of the Evil Obesity Monster. You can find out how many calories are contained in the foods you choose to eat. Buy a book. on amazon or Google, the USDA calorie chart. The calories in restaurant foods are listed on their websites. Practice "Defensive (Dining Ch. 37). Knowledge is Power.

159. Nutritional Awareness

By: Dr. Judith Giustini

What you eat has a major effect on your health, happiness and success. This involves not only how many calories you consume every day, but what nutrients are contained in the foods you choose to eat. Maybe it would have been great if we could have learned this information in grade school and junior high school, but since we probably did not, what can we do about it now? 6 out of 10 of the major causes of death in the U.S. are linked to nutrition, so nutrition would be good to know about.

The recommended daily allowance for all vitamins and minerals is available online, or there are books. Natural foods – fruits and vegetables, beans, etc. are nutritionally dense nutrition. Fragmented foods – sugar, white flour, etc. contain empty calories that require nutrients from the "good" foods to be processed in your metabolism. Water is vital to the functioning of every cell in your body. Your digestive system, your cardiovascular system and your brain are big users of water. One reason for weight gain is dehydration, where the person mistakes thirst for hunger, so they eat when they should be drinking water.

Even if you know every RDA and every nutrient in every food, that does not mean you are going to choose to eat and drink those things your body needs. Maybe you eat what you eat because you like what you like. Maybe you are super-busy and shopping for groceries and preparing nutritious meals for yourself is less convenient than the drive-thru window. Maybe sugar is a regular part of your calories. This is something to consider, because sugar is now being implicated in high cholesterol and high blood pressure, as well as diabetes.

160. Super Soup – Very Veggie

By: Dr. Judith Giustini

1 quart chopped onions
1 head garlic, chopped
1 quart chopped celery
1 quart chopped carrots
1 quart chopped broccoli
1 quart chopped zucchini
2 bags frozen chopped string beans
½ cup olive oil
1 lb. brown rice, cooked with sea salt
1 lb. black beans, cooked with sea salt
1- 2 large can tomato sauce
optional: 1-2 packets onion soup mix

Preheat large cooking pot over high heat
Add olive oil (120 cal. per Tbs.) and onions.
Cook, stirring occasionally until partially cooked
Add carrots, cover and cook for about 10 minutes, stirring occasionally.
When carrots are partially cooked,
The temp should be quite high at this point
Add the other vegetables, except zucchini
Add tomato sauce, plus enough water to cover vegetables
Cook until mixture barely comes to a boil
Add zucchini. Turn off heat.
Wait ½ hour for vegetables to finish cooking
Add rice, beans and bean juice if any
You may need to add some water now.

161. The Super Shakes Plan

By: Dr. Judith Giustini

Fortunately, there is an easy way for you to switch to a diet of fresh raw fruits and vegetables that is delicious and easy to prepare if you have a blender. Amazon has quite a few blenders for less than $50 each. Maybe you will need one for work, or maybe you will need a thermos for when you are out and about.

Recipe: In your blender jar, place a raw apple (65-100 cal.), cut in quarters, with the skin and seeds (just remove the stem and that little rosette at the bottom), an orange (45-86 cal.), with skin and seeds, cut in pieces, a banana (50-100 cal.). Add milk (1% = 103 cal./8 oz., 2% = 122 cal./8 oz., or whole = 149 cal./8 oz.). You might want to add some a no-calorie sweetener such as Stevia, which is made from a plant.

Whiz this up on your blender and see how delicious it is. Maybe sometimes you will want to add a carrot (55 cal.) or some celery (15 cal. per stick). What about summer squash? (1med. 68 cal.), raspberries (1 cup 64 cal.)., pineapple (¼ 115 cal.), (pinto beans (½ cup cooked 99 cal.), cooked sweet potato (1 cup 114 cal.) (See Ch. 169. Calorie Content of Foods).

The Super Shakes Plan contains 4 eggs per day. You can put them in your Super Shakes ("Pasteurized" eggs are okay raw) or make a couple of meals of them (remember, oils are100 cal. per Tbs.). Eggs contain about 75 cal. each, and they are packed with nutrients (Ch. 154.), so they provide "satiety" – a feeling of being satisfied. Maybe you would like to make a meal of 2 eggs, plus a big serving of Stir-Fry (Ch. 165.).

162. Implementing the Super Shakes Plan

By: Dr. Judith Giustini

The goal of The Super Shakes Plan is to supply your body with as much nutrient-dense nutrition as possible within the limits of the number of calories you are allowed to consume each day and lose about 2 lbs. per week, which calories are: 1,200 calories per day for a woman or 1,500 calories per day for a man. Because of your prior excesses with food and drink, you now have some pounds or kilos to lose. This might take "a while", so you need a relatively painless Plan you can stick to.

Your Super Shakes will contain 4 eggs per day, milk, all fruits, some vegetables, (such as squash and sweet potatoes), brown rice, and beans. You may also want to add nutrient powders such as Spirulina, Hemp Seed, Kale or others (amazon). These shakes are delicious, and you will look forward to your next glassful, but you won't go around hungry in the meantime. Maybe you will lose your extra weight, only to find it creeping up again after you go off the Super Shakes Plan. You won't mind doing The Super Shakes Plan again if you need to.

Dining out can be a challenge. You need to practice "Defensive Dining" (Ch. 37). In a sit-down restaurant, maybe you can order a salad and a baked potato or a vegetarian platter of whatever vegetables they are serving that day. In Chinese restaurants or carryout, you can choose steamed brown rice with vegetables, and resist the temptation to nibble on choices from the put-up platter or your friends' dishes. Fast food places publish the calorie content of their menu items on their websites and sometimes inside the restaurants. It's easy to overeat and impede your weight loss progress. Take charge of things in your life.

Google says that in the U.S. 69% of adults are obese, in India, 40.3%, and in China, 48.9%. Many people attribute this situation to the easy availability of high-calorie foods at the drive-thru.

163. How About a Stir-Fry?

By: Dr. Judith Giustini

A Stir-Fry is a meal you can make for yourself or serve to guests. You can use fresh or frozen vegetables and cooked brown rice and boneless skinless chicken breast (maybe from your freezer). Remember that olive oil contains about 120 calories per Tbs. Maybe you could add some vegetable broth or chicken broth to blend the ingredients.

Wash all the vegetables and chop them into small pieces. Heat up a large non-stick frying pan (maybe a wok?), over high heat, add the oil and chopped onions. When they are about cooked, add the garlic and stir for a few minutes. Add the vegetables, starting with those that take longest to cook. Add the rest of the vegetables little by little, and towards the end, add the brown rice (and chopped chicken breast, if desired). Add the broth, if needed, and you're done. Maybe you would like some soy sauce with this.

You can keep some servings of Stir-Fry in your refrigerator and/or freezer. Maybe you can bring some to work and re-heat it for lunch, even share with a work-mate. Note: Ch. 169. is Calorie Content of Foods.

164. Major Weight Loss Company Getting into the Booming Weight Loss Drug Business

By: Dr. Judith Giustini

This month (July, 2023) news stories on NPR and PBS said that Weight Watchers (WW International) has purchased a company named Sequence, which provides a service that links patients with physicians that prescribe weight loss and diabetes drugs via tele-talk.

Some side-effects of weight loss drugs are: increased blood pressure and heart rate, insomnia, nervousness, restlessness, and dependence on and abuse of the drugs.

The original Weight Watchers diet was relatively simple: 1,200 calories for women and 1,500 calories for men, using portion-controlled meals of regular foods, 2 Tbs. butter or oil, 3 fruits per day, etc. Over time, they have added menu items and a points system, plus foods they sell, and they send emails to potential members, advertising that WW meetings are inexpensive now.

Question: If this diet was helping people live in normal-weight bodies, why would they need to take pills suppress their appetite?

Problem: Many people are fat because of overeating "fragmented/overly-processed foods, empty calories and foods from the Drive-Thru window. Maybe their weight has crept up to "enormous" on this diet, but they are kind of addicted to it and they don't see their way out. Their bodies are starving because they are not getting the nutrients they need. (Many of us have done the WW diet and reached goal weight, but it is not a diet we would like to return to, because we felt hungry much of the time.)

165. Why Did You Get Fat?

By: Dr. Judith Giustini

Maybe you have Lack of Knowledge – you don't know how many calories you can consume each day without gaining weight, so you eat what you eat because you like what you like. An adult woman requires about 2,000 calories per day; an adult man requires about 2,500 calories per day.

On the Classic Weight-Loss diet of 1,200/1,500 calories per day, you will lose about 2 lbs. per week. If you just get a calorie chart and check out the calories of each food you consume, you can develop "Calorie Consciousness". If you stay on this course, you may develop "Nutritional Awareness" and make better choices.

Maybe your life is very busy – work, school, family, etc. -too busy to try a diet, or you are in poor health, too weak to try a diet. Maybe you are upset about your obesity, and you keep berating yourself and judging yourself harshly and this drives you to the cookie jar.

Maybe **your Fat** is linked to feelings of a need for protection, resistance to forgiving, or hidden anger.

Maybe you have subconscious negative feelings related to adverse childhood (or other) experiences. (See: AOO126. Mind-Body Therapy vs. Obesity)

166. Feelings Associated with Obesity
From: Feelings Buried Alive Never Die

By: Karol K. Truman – by Dr. Judith Giustini

By: Dr. Judith Giustini

Fat:

Feel a need for protection
Resistance to forgiving Hidden anger

Obesity:

Using food as a substitute for affection
Inability to admit to others what you truly desire
Inability to express your feelings
Seeking love
Protecting the body
Trying to fulfill the self
Stuffed feelings
A feeling of power and a desire to throw one's weight around

Over-Eating (compulsive):

Tension
Feeling a material-emotional lack
Craving closeness
Putting on emotional armor
Emotional energy based on anger & resentment

Overweight

> Feelings of insecurity
> Feelings of self-rejection
> Wanting to protect the body
> Seeking love & fulfillment
> Feelings are stuffed inside

167. Calories in Foods from Internet research

By: Dr. Judith Giustini

For complete listing, you can get a USDA calorie chart online, or order a book from amazon. Most restaurant chains post the calorie content of their menu items on their websites.

FRUITS:

Apple	1 (28.35 g)	95 cal
Apricot	1 (35 g)	17 cal
Banana	1 (125 g)	111 cal
Cantaloupe	Wedge (69 g)	23 cal
Lemon	1 (58 g)	17 cal
Orange	1 (131 g)	62 cal
Peach	1 (150 g)	59 cal
Pineapple	1 (905 g)	453 cal
Plum	1 (66 g)	30 cal
Raspberries	1 cup (123 g	64 cal

VEGETABLES

Bean Sprouts	1 portion	48 cal
Beets, canned	1 cup	29 cal
Bell pepper	1 cup	35 cal
Broccoli	1 cup	68 cal
Carrots	1 cup	100 cal
Cauliflower	1cup	66 cal
Celery	1 cup	27 cal
Cucumber	1 slice	1 cal
Eggplant	300 g	59 cal
Green beans	200 g	79 cal

Green peas	25 g	23 cal
Kale	100 g	43 cal
Onions	1 medium	44 cal
Radish	15 g	3 cal
Red Cabbage	200 g	55 cal
Squash, yellow	1 medium	68 cal
Squash, Zucchini	1 medium	33 cal
Sweet Potato	1 cup cubes	114 cal

BEANS & RICE

Lentils cooked	1 cup	230 cal
Pinto beans	½ cup cooked	99 cal
Brown rice	1 cup cooked	216 cal

EGGS, MILK, CHICKEN

Egg	1 egg (50 g)		78 cal
Whole milk	1 cup		150 cal
	2% milk	1 cup	122 cal
	1% milk	1 cup	106 cal
	Skim milk	1 cup	84 cal

Chicken breast1 boneless, skinless   284 cal

CALORIES IN McDONALD'S FOODS

Hamburger	250 cal
Cheeseburger	300 cal
Big Mac	590 cal
Quarter Pounder	520-630 cal
Egg McMuffin	290 cal
Sesame Sausage Egg Bagel	610 cal
Hotcakes with syrup and butter	550 cal
Vanilla milk shake, medium	570 cal

168. What You Breathe as a Cause of Stress

By: Dr. Judith Giustini

These days (2024), there is a trend toward "green" – where many governments are investing in solar and wind as energy sources for electricity, however, there is also a worldwide increase of coal in power plants. People (especially children who live near coal-burning often have lung problems. Soldiers who lived near "burn pits" have are being treated in veterans' hospitals. Many first responders at the World Trade Center Disaster on September 11, 2001 have had ongoing lung illnesses and some people still smoke tobacco.

In the 1940's and 1950's cigarette advertising was in magazines and newspapers and on billboards. Cigarette vending machines were conveniently located. People could smoke in bars and restaurants. In the 1960's came the lawsuits against tobacco companies and the Surgeon General report: SMOKING IS HAZARDOUS TO YOUR HEALTH.

If What You Breathe is cigarette smoke, it is a cause of stress because a harsh poison that can cause lung cancer and predispose you (like obesity) to other illnesses. It is a cause of stress because you are addicted, and it makes your teeth turn yellow and it makes you stink. How about the expense! Cigarettes now cost about $7.50 per pack ($.25 per pack in the 1960's).

How to Quit Smoking Tobacco: (1) DECIDE TO QUIT. (2) Choose a time when you have 3 to stay home. (3) See if you can get some meds to help you sleep through the ordeal. (4) Assemble treats you like: candy, ice cream, foods -whatever. (5) Prepare to watch movies and videos. (6) QUIT. After 48 hours, the craving will be much less, and after 60 hours, it should be gone. (7) DO NOT "try" to smoke a cigarette to see if it makes you dizzy.

169. Restaurant Chains Closing Locations 2023-2024

By: Dr. Judith Giustini

A Google search in April, 2024 listed:

Cracker Barrel
Applebee's
Krispy Kreme
Boston Market
TGI Fridays
Pizza Hut
Burger King
Red Lobster
Ruby Tuesday
PDQ
Denny's
Taco Bueno
and Mod Pizza
Outback Steakhouse
Carrabba's Italian Grill
Bonefish Grill
Tijuana Flats

as companies going out of business or closing many locations. for various reasons.

170. A Little Final Note

By: Dr. Judith Giustini

You may have noticed that the chapters of this book could be in a better sequential order. 20 years ago, they were in alphabetical order, but then they developed some friends and relations, and they ended up where they are now.

The purpose of this book is to inform you and support you in your journey to living in a normal-weight body – to hold your hand and encourage you. Even if you only read one page (chapter) per day, it can keep your mind on your goal, and help you take charge of things in your life.

I am looking to do videos of myself reading each chapter to you, and posting them on my new website, so that if you are feeling distracted or confused, or you just don't feel like reading, you can click and find somebody to read it to you.

My other book is *Mind-Body Therapy and Your Health, Happiness, and Success.* If you are a healthcare professional, it can be a doorway to a new modality that can bring you joy to and enhance your practice.

- I am looking to start a Zoom School and maybe a YouTube channel.

Contact info: Dr. Judith Giustini

> 1100 Main Street
> Danville, VA 24541
> mindbodytherapist60@gmail.com
> mindbodytherapist.net

We can arrange a time if you would like to schedule an initial free chat.